Voyage: A Beginner's Guide to Paleo
London Solomon

**Cookbook and Workbook,
the first of many products brought to you by Felicity.**

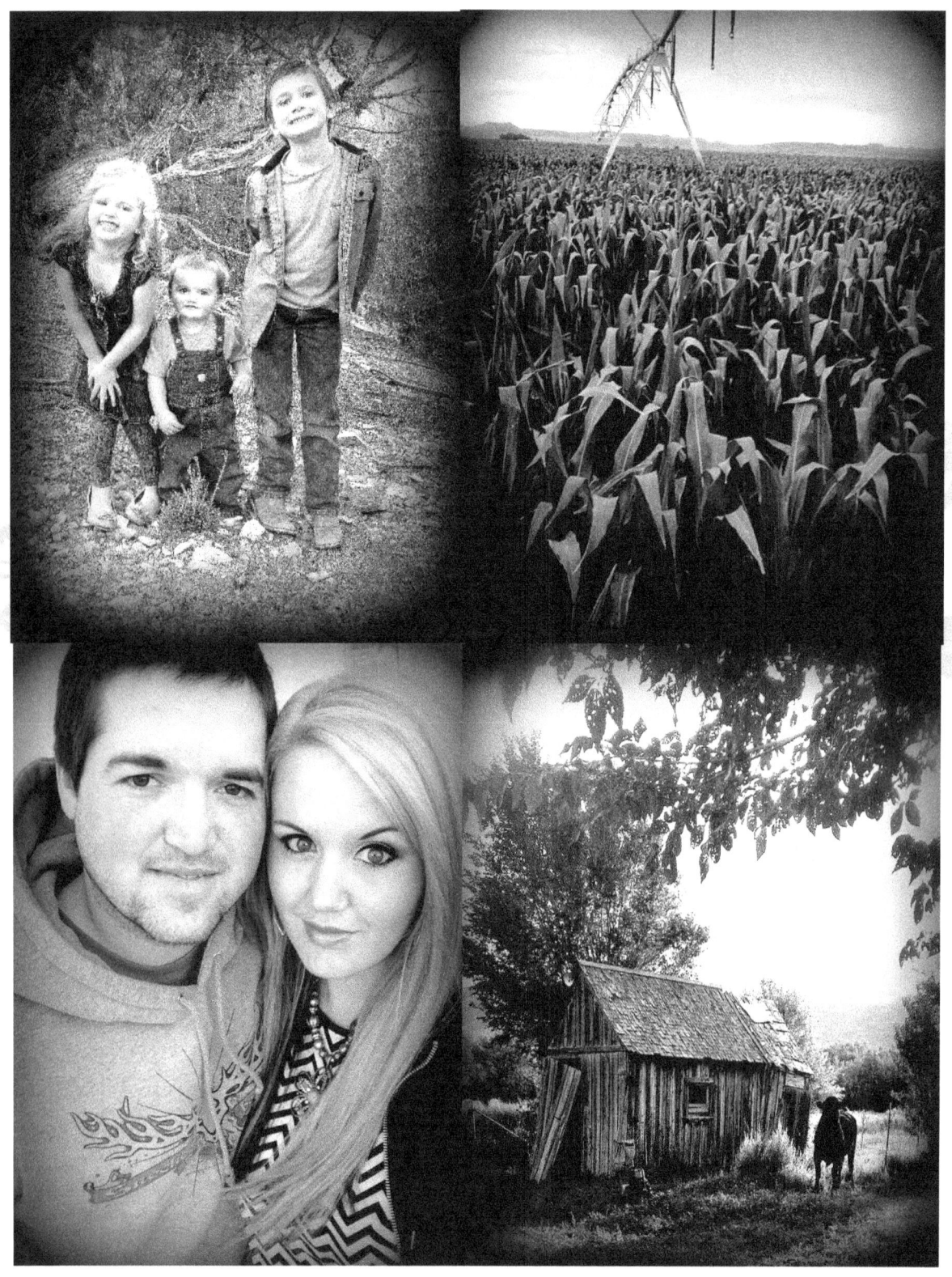

Dedication

For my Father in Heaven
and his son, my savior, Jesus Christ.

For my beloved husband, Eric.
You are the love of my life.
You taught me to love and laugh again.
You believed in me when no one else did.
You loved me when I couldn't love myself.
Thank you for coming along with me on this journey.
Thank you for your unconditional support.
Thank you for loving me like only you do.
I would've never tried, if not for you.
Wherever you go, I'll be by your side.
For with you I am complete…
and I am home.

For Kelson, Kaylee, and Grant.
There are no words that could justly express the way every ounce of my soul loves you.
I wouldn't be the woman I am today if not for the opportunity to be your mother.
You are my greatest source of strength, inspiration, and a beaming light—
even in the darkest of worlds.
Someday I hope you are as proud to be my children, as I am to be your mommy.

For my grandfather, Grant Messerly.
I hope heaven is full of bouncing baby lambs and a heart full of pride for the legacy you left behind.

Special Thanks To:

Dr. Terrence Heath,
You started this all. You saved me.

Ashlee Hoyle,
Without your editing work and encouragement, I may have never found the courage to publish.

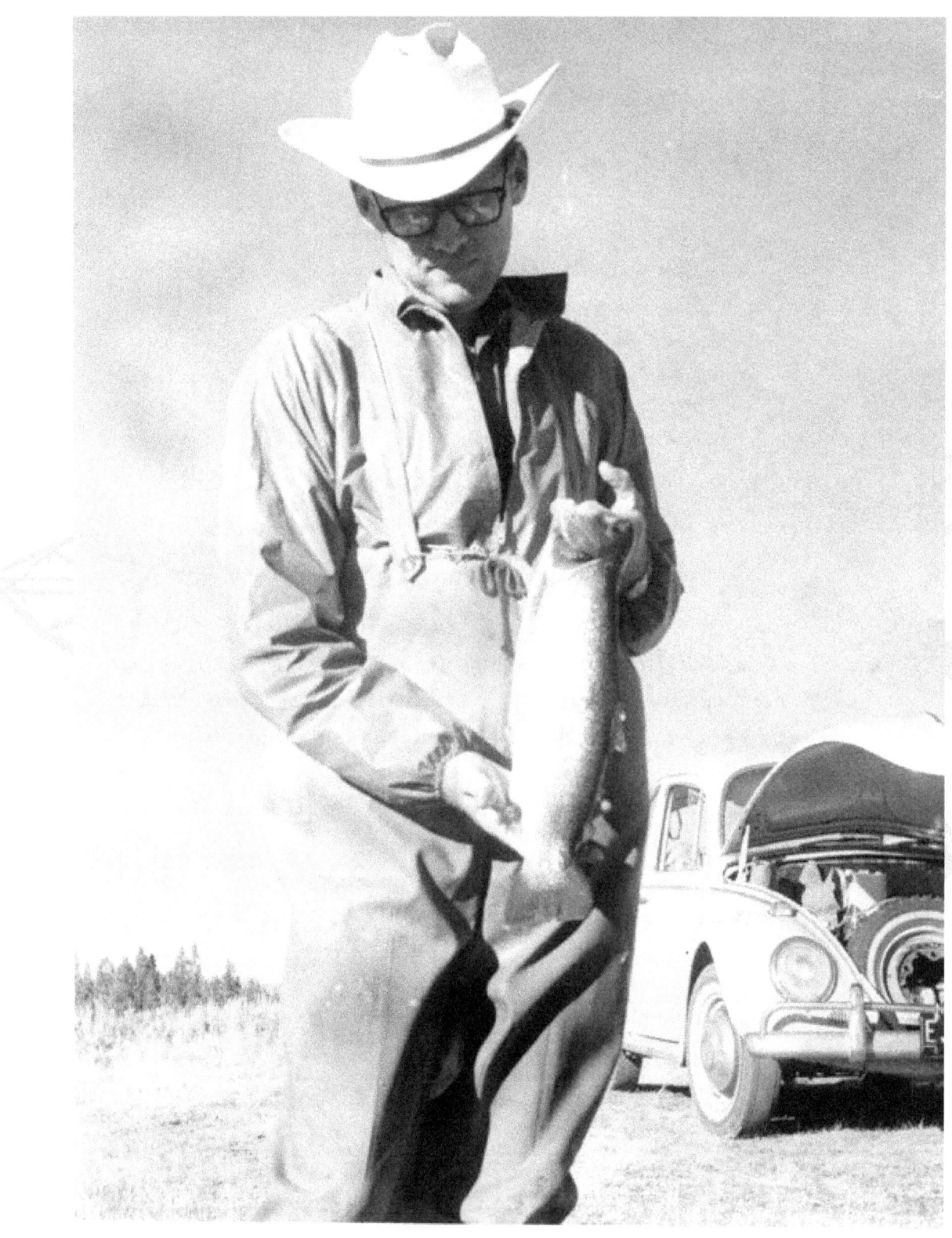

Index

Recipes

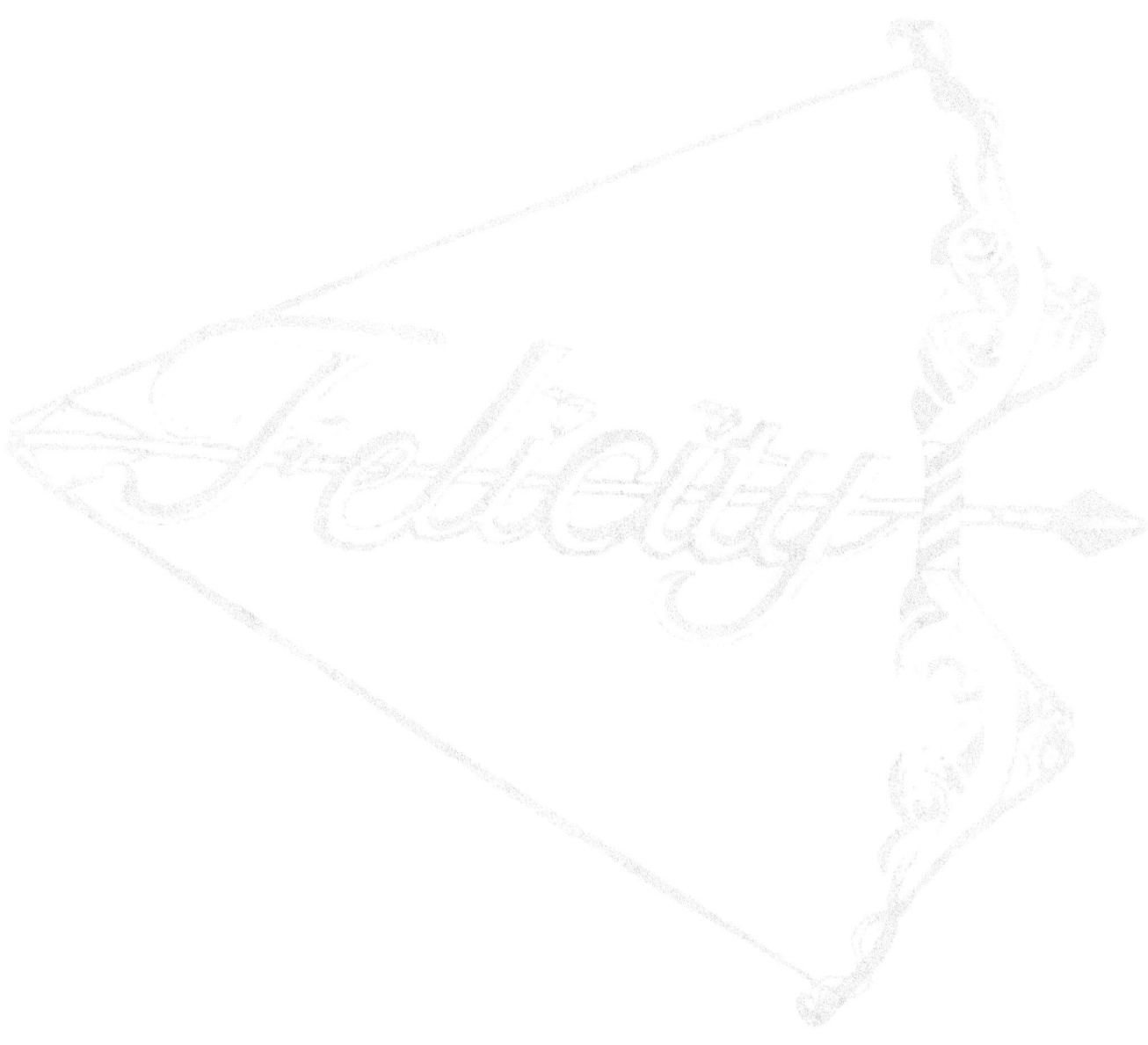

Finding Felicity

Have you ever watched as a child danced through a field of wildflowers?
Have you ever listened to a little girl laugh out loud at the chirping birds in the sky?
Have you ever seen the crooked smile of a child who has just captured a grasshopper?
Have you ever wondered how children can run and run and run but they never tire?
Have you ever thought that children look like angels, floating just above the ground?

This is because their spirits are not tied down to society's complex definitions
of good and bad, beautiful and ugly, or even right and wrong.
They smile, laugh, and dance around without a care in the world.
Children are inherently free.
We are all born free.

Those who refuse to conform to the pressures of worldly expectations
remain free throughout their lives.

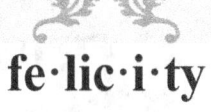

fe·lic·i·ty

noun

1. intense happiness.
"domestic felicity"
2. the ability to find appropriate
expression for one's thoughts. "speech
that pleased by its accuracy, felicity,
and fluency"

About the Author

London Solomon

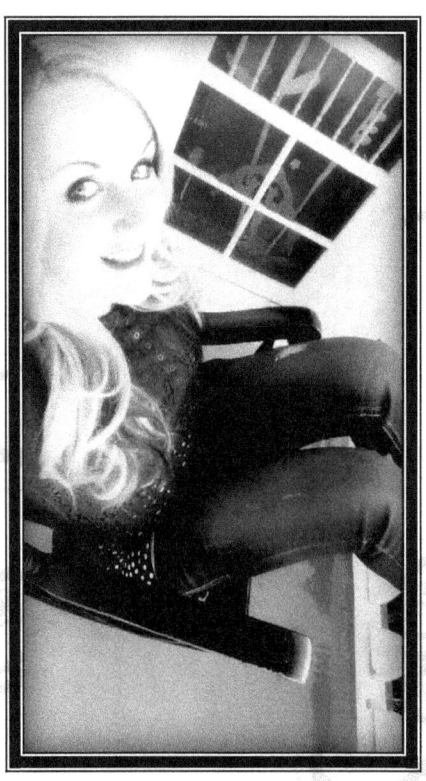

I'd like to tell you a little about myself. My name is London Solomon. I am not a nutritionist. I am not a personal trainer. I am not ashamed to admit that I am a woman who has spent most of my life battling mental illness. There is a stigma attached to mental illness in society that I am bound and determined to destroy, but that is another cause for another day.

I am a woman. I am a writer and a creator. I am a mother and I am a wife. At one time, I was a little girl who hated herself. Looking back, I don't remember any point in my life that I didn't hate my body. I have always been very tall, and I vividly remember wishing I could be the same size as all of the other girls in my elementary school classes. Even in the sweet innocence of childhood, I was plagued with self-hate. As far back as the kindergarten, I remember desperately hating myself. I have spent most my life suffering from clinical depression, crippling anxiety, hormonal imbalances, severe body dysmorphic disorder, and later in life these illnesses progressed into severe eating disorders and a death grip that only addiction can hold on your soul. After many years of trying everything possible to escape the private, personal hell that I had trapped myself in, I finally found the cure to my soul's illnesses through the Paleo lifestyle.

I will discuss the practice of a Paleo diet later in the book, but first I feel that I need to take readers and myself back to the basics, back to my childhood, where I learned everything I needed to know about life. This journey of reflection is not an easy one. I lost my way for many years. This book is not the end of my story, but a detailed account of my journey towards finding me and my own personal felicity.

Voyage: London's Voyage
London Solomon

To Fly

There is an unseen majestic wonder down dirt roads in small towns. No words describe the euphoria one can feel as their feet beat against a hidden dirt road that only exists because the powerful forces beneath the hood of a rumbling tractor, driven by a farmer headed off to work during dawn, passed through. As your legs move faster and you begin to feel stronger than you ever have, it is as if the weight of the world falls from your soul with every earth pounding leap. There are no struggles. There is no sadness, no anger, and no pain. There is just simple, calm nothingness when you allow yourself to become one with nature.

This practice is not exercise.
It is not about physical strength or endurance.
One's body is capable of miraculous strength when the soul is let free.
It is religion.
It is *my religion*.
It is as close to heaven as we, on earth, can come.
It is the ultimate source of spiritual strength.

This experience can be so empowering that the human body cannot keep up the flying soul and one cannot help but collapse ... but it doesn't matter. It doesn't hurt as you fall into the earth because you are there.

You have met divine *Felicity.*

The peace and spiritual calmness that one can find while lying in at the edge of a green field, watching the sun rest behind a mountain as another day comes to an end, is the purest level of serenity I have ever known. The world is full of beauty and chances to become one with nature. As with all miracles, finding personal enlightenment through nature takes one's time and undivided attention. Most chances are missed because we are too busy to stop and notice.

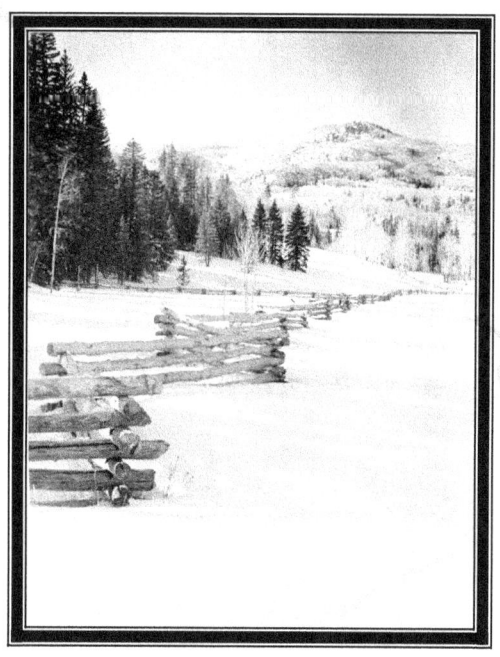

Dirt

I spent my childhood covered, head to toe, in Southern Utah dirt. I enjoyed the innocence of simple country living in a very small town. The most valuable lessons I learned were not taught to me in a classroom, but while climbing through bales of hay and standing, with my beloved cousins and siblings, on the edge of fences peering through the cracks of old wood and watching as a simple old man dedicated all of himself to his farm, his family, and his sheep.

We watched from the sidelines as he built a legacy that we have spent our adult lives understanding, appreciating, and cherishing memories of simpler times. I was shown, by old beautiful souls, just what the good life is.

Spring time meant lambing season and my spring months were spent with my brothers and cousins. We didn't know it then, but we were in the heart of the circle of life as we hung around the sheds eagerly awaiting the arrival of new baby lambs. Looking back, I am realizing that the experience of watching the miracle of new life in the birth of lambs, as a young child, was the foundation that I built my life upon. My childhood was sweet. My grandfather was a stern, strong man, but there were so many simple, tender moments that he taught us all how to love with unwavering sincerity. I witnessed God's work in saving lost sheep on the mountain where they grazed. I learned to nurture the ill and less fortunate while bottle feeding orphaned lambs. I felt the tender heartache of loss as I held a baby lamb in my arms while its life slipped away. I learned that death was an inevitable piece of the circle of life, and although painful for those of us left behind, somehow I came to the understanding that death could be as beautiful as birth. Both are just a transaction of souls. I watched souls come into to the world, and I watched some leave, but I am certain that all lambs go to heaven.

Perhaps, only I perceived the process this way. Maybe my childish mind couldn't comprehend loss yet - I don't know. What I do know is that this understanding of life and death has brought peace to me in the face of tragedy later in life. Through years of diligently observing my grandfather, I learned that the most intelligent people search for their soul's passion and when they find it, no matter where life takes them, they stay true to themselves. I learned the value of a hard day's work and that if I wanted respect, I'd damn well be ready to earn it and prove myself or get out of the way. I learned that a man is only as good as his word is true. I learned that sunshine is the best medicine. I learned that no family is perfect, regardless, you take care of those who belong to you, and that the strongest men take the time to show their grandchildren how to tenderly love all living creatures.

Every day, my brother and I crawled out of bed before the sun to deliver the newspaper to the people who lived in our town. We saddled up our horses and rode around this quiet little town, carelessly tossing the rolled up Spectrum newspaper into our neighbors' yards. I hated waking up so early, but the sunrise took my breath away every single day. The most precious time of my youth was spent in the mountains where I felt most at home on the back of my old paint mare. She was my best friend, and at times my only companion. She offered an unconditional sense of acceptance that I longed for because I couldn't accept myself. The rhythmic sound her hooves made as they met the earth was the musical soundtrack of my innocence.

My memories are vivid and so very precious but somewhere, in the midst of life's chaos and the process of "growing up," I forgot the soul healing power of dirt roads.

The Tiny Hands Hold My Soul

I often find myself wondering what I did to make God believe that I deserved the blessing of my three beautiful children. They, and my husband, are the loves of my life. They hold my heart in their tiny, often dirty, fingers.

Kelson, Kaylee, and Grant are the best pieces of me.
My incredibly intelligent son, Kelson, is 8 years old.
My bouncy beautiful daughter, Kaylee, is 5 years old.
My sweet little baby boy, Grant, is 2 years old.

I found out that Kelson was on his way a few short weeks before my high school graduation. The moment he entered this world, I knew I could not live my life apart from him. It didn't matter that I was still a child myself, he was mine and I was his. Heaven sent my beautiful little angel, Kaylee, two short years later. I found myself left to figure out how to be a mother, all on my own. The three of us had to grow up together. We learned our own lessons, many of which were figured out the hard way. Nothing ever came easy for us but even with the odds stacked against us, we learned to appreciate the beauty of the simplicity that was our world.

In the early years of their lives, I discovered a love like nothing I had ever imagined. They were so pure, so strong, and so innocent. I often say that my children and I share an old hippy's soul. They find the same solitude in nature that I always have. We spent our days at home down by the river casting stones and laughing as the ripples turned to waves. Life hasn't always been easy, but there was always beauty to be found.

I would like to express my deepest gratitude for your interest in my life transformation and my journey to finding Felicity. I chose the name "Felicity" for my company because it best describes what, I believe, everyone spends their lives searching for, ***intense happiness***.

> *"The secret of health for both mind and body is not to mourn for the past, worry about the future, or anticipate troubles, but to live in the present moment wisely and earnestly."*

To Rebuild

Shortly after giving birth to my third child, I was struggling to balance my family life with the addition of my beautiful new baby and a devastating diagnosis of my oldest son I knew that I couldn't go on like this. I walked into my OB's office in tears about my weight and uncontrollable depression. I was there to desperately beg that he give me antidepressants. This is when he first introduced me to the idea of a Paleo lifestyle. I am more grateful than words can say for this wonderful man and for his advice, compassion, and guidance. He will never understand how he has forever changed the broken woman I used to be.

He sat down beside me and explained how properly nourishing our bodies can help self-regulate our hormones, potentially balancing themselves out which will relieve physical and psychological symptoms brought on by improper nutrition. I was skeptical as he began writing on a prescription pad. Never could I have known that three little lines would forever change the woman I am. He wrote,

"No sugar.
No grains.
No dairy."

I had nothing left of myself to lose.

I was faced with the horrifying realization that my first born child was autistic, and in my current state I felt I was not equipped or worthy of being his mother or anyone's mother. Perhaps it was my inexperience, my young age, or just the fact that I was incapable of seeing flaw in a perfect child, but when my oldest son was diagnosed with Autism Spectrum Disorder, I broke. I completely lost myself.

Autism

November 20th, 2013

That was the day everything changed forever. That was the day that my greatest fears were confirmed. My beautiful child was officially diagnosed with autism spectrum disorder. I was hit with a wave of emotions, fear and failure being the most prevalent. I sat down that evening and wrote because it was all I had left. I had to somehow get this overwhelming sense of grief out of my body, and the only way I knew to do that was to write. Below are the unpolished words I wrote that evening, through an uncontrollable stream of burning hot tears, as I tried to comprehend where I would find the strength to be the mother he would need throughout his life.

Angry. This morning I woke up and I was so angry. No, not angry... Furious, hateful, irate ... My alarm went off, I kept my eyes shut. I wasn't going to open them. Kelson wasn't awake yet. He didn't need to go to school. We'd just sleep in. We'd just hide from the world today. We'd just pretend nothing was wrong with anyone. We'd just pretend that everything was just fine. You see, I got a phone call last night informing me that all of Kelson's testing had been "scored" and the school psychologist is now ready to "go over it" with me. This morning I was weak. I didn't care. I turned off my alarm, covered my face with my blankets, I rocked myself back and forth, I cried and cried and cried. I tried my hardest to fall back asleep but I couldn't escape the ugliness in my head. I thought;

Maybe if I hadn't been so young ... Kelson wouldn't have autism.

Maybe if I had focused more on Kelson and less on my own education, Kelson wouldn't have autism.

Maybe if I hadn't worked so hard ... Maybe if I had worked harder ... Kelson wouldn't have autism.

Maybe if I had more money or more time ... Kelson wouldn't have autism.

Maybe if I hadn't been "too tired," "too stressed," "too busy" ... Kelson wouldn't have autism.

Maybe if I didn't have 2 more kids ... Kelson wouldn't have autism.

Maybe if I had been more stable and moved less ... Kelson wouldn't have autism.

Maybe if I had breastfed him ... Or maybe if I hadn't vaccinated him... Kelson wouldn't have autism.

Maybe if I hadn't spent so many years hating God ... Kelson wouldn't have autism.

Maybe if I hadn't been so weak ... Kelson wouldn't have autism.

Maybe if I had been a better mother ... Kelson wouldn't have autism.

Maybe if I hadn't been so selfish ... Maybe if I'd given him up for adoption (like so many suggested I do) to a more deserving, loving, and prepared mother ... Kelson wouldn't have autism.

Maybe Kelson doesn't have autism ... No, maybe if I hadn't been in denial for so long ... Kelson wouldn't have autism.

All emotional irrationality aside, it didn't much matter this morning. What was done was done and here we were, finally being forced to face this long awaited "judgment day." I had envisioned the day that an actual diagnosis was made being a day that we sat down and outlined all the mistakes I have made as a mother, a day where I promised that I had matured and that I am a much better mother than I used to be, and a day that would negatively define my innocent child for the rest of his life. A part of me hoped that I was making it all up, that I would walk in there and the psychologist would roll his eyes and tell me that I am being overdramatic; my child is absolutely fine … I guess I knew that wasn't going to happen though.

Moving along. Kelson got up at about 9 and came into my bedroom dressed and ready to go to school. I drug myself out of bed, got the little kids dressed, and strapped them all into the car. I drove slower than usual. I wasn't ready. I tapped the breaks a few times as we passed several little dirt roads that I seriously considered turning down, just to avoid going to the school. I have driven this road a thousand times but today, it seemed so short. In no time, we were there. Kelson hopped out of the car and walked into the school. I had to take Kaylee and Grant to my mom's house. I wanted so badly to reach out and grab onto him. I wanted to beg him to stay with me! I didn't want him going in there. I was angry. I hated school. I hated psychology. I hated myself. Mostly. I HATED AUTISM! I couldn't see how any of this was fair. I couldn't understand who the hell anyone in that building thought they were or why they thought they had the right to decide who is sick or not sick, who is crazy or not crazy! How dare they "score" my child. How dare they judge him, me, US!

Once I finally returned to the school for my meeting, my eyes poured tears at the site of the playground. I just wanted him to be normal. I just wanted him to play and bask in the sweet innocence of childhood like I did on that very playground. It wasn't fair. It isn't fair. I nodded my head and quietly whispered the occasional, "Okay… Yeah" as the psychologist went over the test results. It took everything I had to hold in my anger, my hatred for the disorder. Once the word "autism" was finally said out loud, the psychologist gave me a strange look and said,

"You didn't have much of a response to the word, you must have already suspected autism."

I wanted to yell, stomp, and cry… Yes. I had "suspected" it. Yes. I have known for some time that my son was struggling. I tried. I begged. I pleaded. I asked over and over again for help and was repeatedly told, "Wait for kindergarten." I spent an entire summer anxiously awaiting and dreading this very moment. YES! I KNOW MY SON HAS AUTISM BUT FOR SOME ABSURD REASON, SOMEONE HAS TO HEAR IT FROM YOU BEFORE THEY WILL DO A DAMN THING ABOUT IT!

As he went on about the test results, my mind wandered back to a time, 3 or so years ago, that I took my sweet little Kelson to a counselor. I was in the middle of a divorce and Kelson's behavioral problems escalated to an all-time high. He was out of control. Worse though, was that I was out of control. Neither of us could control our emotions or our anger toward the crappy hands we had been dealt. I sat with this counselor and Kelson for an hour talking about the problems we were having. She had no answers. She offered no advice. She walked me out to my car and Kelson started one of his tantrums because he didn't want to buckle into his car seat. She smirked and I so vividly remember watching the words, "I don't know what you are going to do. All I know is that he is never going to be an easy child" come out of her mouth.

Today, after finally getting through the most difficult conversation that I have had to have in my entire life, I have only 2 words for the counselor who saw Kelson and I 3 years ago, SCREW YOU! He is not a "difficult child." He is not damaged and neither am I. He is going to get through this. He is going to be something great because there are good, caring people in the world who are watching out for him now. As hard as this day has been, I am more grateful than ever for the Iron County School District and Escalante Valley Elementary. FINALLY someone is here to help us. Tonight, I may feel just as lost as I did this morning but it is so nice to know that I am no longer alone in this battle.

The term "autism" still leaves a bitter taste in my mouth and a soreness in my heart. He doesn't deserve this. It isn't fair. Life just isn't fair sometimes. But he is alive. He is strong, healthy, and happy. He is my hero. My tiny, knight in shining armor because tonight, as I tried SO hard to hold in the tears that wouldn't stop coming; he held my hand, looked into my eyes, giggled a little, and said,

"LET'S TURN THAT FROWN UPSIDE DOWN AND MAKE A MUSIC BIDEO (video)"

… so tonight, the evening following the day that my deepest fears were confirmed, we made a music video to Lady Gaga's *Born This Way*.

Someday, I will look back on this day and I won't remember the terror, the anxiety, the anger. I will remember the way we danced… how we laughed… and laughed … and laughed …

It wasn't about me anymore but I was still sick.

I took my OB's advice and fell in love with myself for the first time in my entire life. It wasn't easy. I had to fight like hell to save myself so I could save my son. There were moments I failed, there were moments I was weak, and times that I wanted to give up. Paleo was not a diet for me, it was a lifestyle. I had to change the way I viewed food, myself, and understand that what I chose to put into my body could either fuel and strengthen me physically, emotionally, and spiritually or cause me to continue to suffer from my lifelong battle with self-hate.

If not for the Paleo lifestyle, I don't know that I would have survived his first year of kindergarten. I had to change. I couldn't afford to hate myself. I couldn't afford to be weak.These beautiful little humans were counting on me. I had to be better for them. I had to be braver than my son's autism. I had to be stronger than the debilitating depression that has controlled my life for the last 20 years.

I was at a crossroads - it was a terribly surreal "DO OR DIE" moment in my life.

I decided to DO. I decided to fix myself, once and for all.

Pounding

On an unusually cool evening in May 2014, after I tucked my sweet children into their beds, I sat on my couch and mindlessly stared out my window for a few minutes. It had been a very difficult few weeks in my little world. I was exhausted from the stresses of life, and I suppose my body could no longer endure the pressure that my racing, confused mind had been putting on it. I didn't usually go out to walk at night, but that evening I found myself lacing up my tennis shoes and heading out my backdoor. It was almost as if my body was taking me somewhere my mind had no interest in going, but I couldn't stop it. I walked down the street, unsure of where I was headed.

My feet started moving faster. I was running. I ran and ran and ran. The pain radiating up my legs, which had weakened over the years, was not enough to stop them from pushing further and further. Harder and harder. I wondered if I would be able to stop them as I turned down a dirt road that ran alongside a field that was glowing beneath the shining sun. My feet pounded against the earth so hard that I could feel the vibration behind my eyes. I wondered if I were shaking the world beneath me. I couldn't breathe but I couldn't stop and I didn't ever want to.

Suddenly my little puppy, that I didn't even realize had tagged along, crossed my path. I swerved to avoid him and my knees became weak from the jolt. I slammed against the rocks and found myself lying face up in the middle of the road staring at the sky. There I was, lying in the dirt; I had not a care in the world. I laughed out loud until my eyes leaked tears.
Then I began to cry. Unexpectedly, I became overwhelmed with emotion. I wasn't even sure what I was crying about, but I was fairly sure that they were tears of joy. I hadn't felt so alive in so many years. I hadn't felt so free since childhood; it was clear to me then that my spirit had been longing for wide open spaces. I pushed up, onto my knees, and thanked God.
I needed to fall down. I needed to laugh. I needed to stop, lie in the dirt, and watch the sunset through sprinkler lines.

I was cold. I was out of breath.

I was free.

I have spent the last two years researching and falling in love with the Paleo lifestyle.

Although I do not practice Paleo 100% of the time, (I follow Paleo 80% of the time and the other 20% consists of some healthy dairy, which I will discuss later) I have personally experienced remarkable physical, emotional, and spiritual benefits from completely transforming my diet and eliminating grains, sugars, and most processed food. Not only have I lost 50+ pounds, but I have learned to love and live again. I have finally freed myself.

I hope that I can help some of you fall in love with life again.

Voyage: Living a Paleo Lifestyle
London Solomon

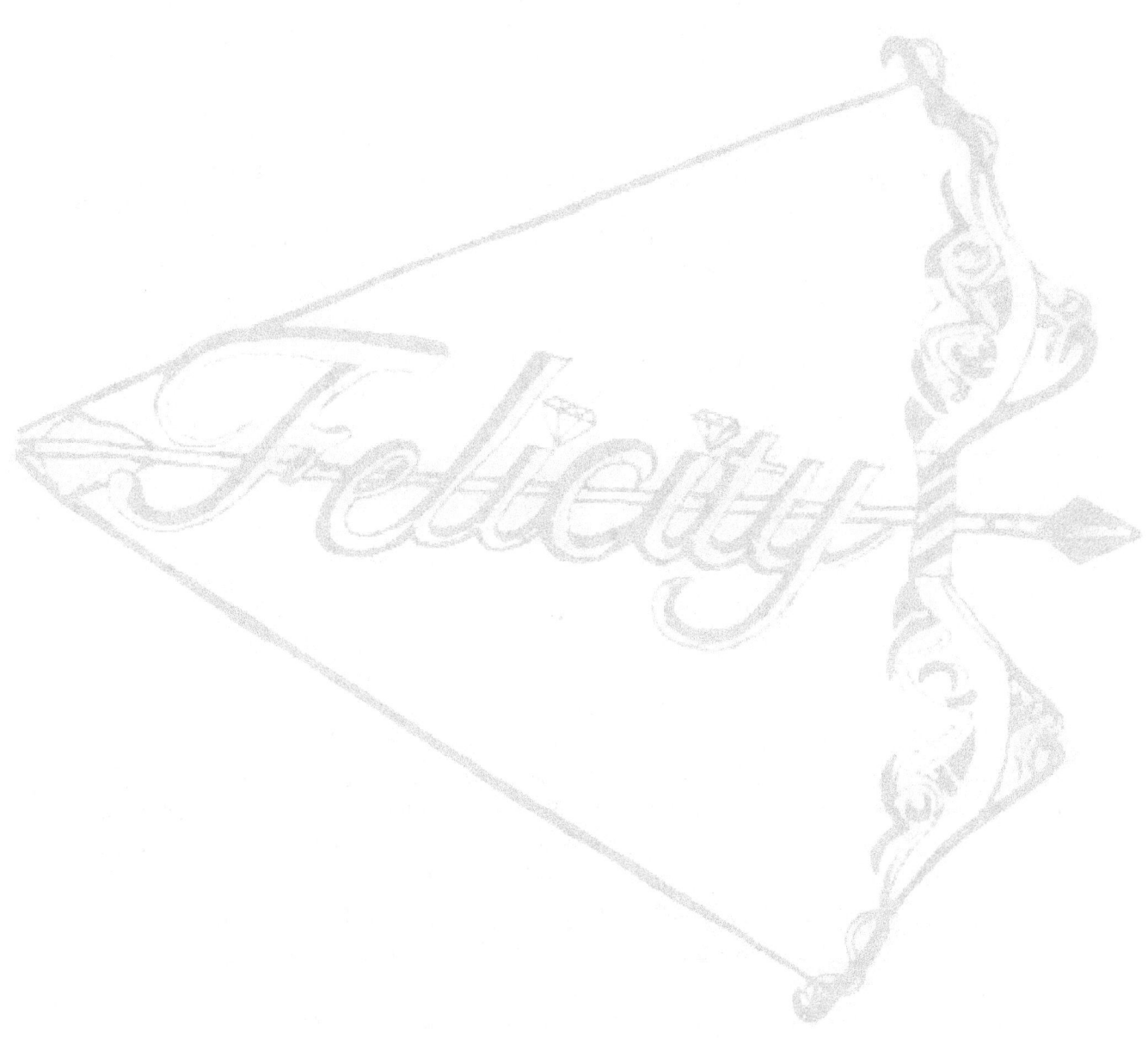

The Basics: Survival

With so many of the food choices that are available being eliminated by saying, "No grains, sugar, or dairy," it is common for people to ask what DOES someone who eats according to the Paleo lifestyle eat. The word "Paleo" is derived from the people who lived in the Paleolithic time era, hunters and gatherers. They ate what the earth offered; they survived off nature. They were lean and strong, a far cry from the millions of people battling obesity around the world. Embrace what is real, what is not manufactured in a plant somewhere. Feed your body foods that will fuel it, rather than weigh it down.

My rule of thumb is this; *if it was born or grew from the earth, eat it.*

The exceptions to this rule are corn, soy, beans, wheat, and potatoes. When eating a Paleo diet, you are choosing foods that will build your body's strength and restore its natural energy. What you WILL eat is plenty of meat, vegetables, fruit, nuts, and healthy fats. These foods will enable your body to heal from injury and illness, you will enjoy a natural burst of energy, and your body will begin shedding unneeded pounds almost immediately.

The Paleo diet is typically low in carbohydrates and high in fat. This does not mean that you will be depriving yourself of carbohydrates. Your body will just be receiving them from sources that it can operate much more efficiently on. Fruit and vegetables are the main source of carbohydrates that you will consume. They contain the vital nutrients that your body needs to function at its highest potential. Before we get too far into exactly what you'll be eating, there are a few practices that you must understand. Turning these few practices in to habit will prove to be just as important, if not more important, than what you feed your body.

Vital Practices to Achieve Your Goals:

1. **Sleep**
   Sleep is the absolute most important aspect of successfully living the Paleo lifestyle. In the beginning, your body will go through a transitioning period as you eliminate the toxic, processed food it has been fed for years. You may even experience a withdrawal period where you feel lethargic and irritable. This is absolutely normal, and although the process (that usually only lasts the first few days but can last up to a week) can be difficult, it is vital to get through the first few days. Studies have shown that sugar and the chemicals used in processed food can be as addictive as cocaine and other drugs. You will literally be reprograming and healing your brain and body. Your body will need sleep, more than ever, as it detoxifies itself and adjusts to your new Paleo lifestyle.
   Do not be discouraged. Once you have broken through the detoxing period, you will experience the most incredible, restful sleep as you continue on your Paleo journey. Your body will begin to self-regulate. You will learn to listen to your body as you begin enjoying natural energy all day and peaceful calmness at night. Make sleep a priority. Make a goal to sleep NO LESS than seven hours at night. Eight to ten hours is ideal.

2. Hydration

Proper hydration is another huge aspect of the Paleo lifestyle. Drinking enough water will play a huge role in the first few days (detox period). Keeping yourself properly hydrated will decrease unhealthy cravings, improve your immune system, lubricate your joints, improve your skin, and aid in healing your digestive system as it flushes toxins out of your system. Making sure that your body receives enough water is as important as what you eat. It should be the first thing you do in the morning and the last thing you do at night. For at least the first week, drink no less than one gallon of water every day. Consume a minimum of 100 ounces of water every day. Do not add flavored drink mixes or any other prepackaged product to your water. I have found, however, that it is easier for me to reach my daily water goal if I add a little sliced cucumber and lemon in my ice water.

You may also drink coffee, herbal teas, and nut milk while following the paleo lifestyle, but these beverages do NOT count towards your daily water goal.

3. Realistic Expectations: Paleo on a Budget

Most traditional Paleo guides and other sources of information place a great level of importance on eating only organic produce and grass-fed meat. Although I am sure that being able to feed yourself and your family only organic and grass-fed food has its benefits, truthfully I wouldn't know. This has never been something that has been possible for my family and our budget. The most common concern expressed to me about beginning a Paleo lifestyle is the cost. Food is expensive. REAL food is even more expensive, and it is not possible for many families, including my own, to live by the standards considered 100% Paleo. In a perfect world, we would feed ourselves and our children organic, homegrown produce. We would all eat only grass-fed, locally slaughtered meat. We can spend all day reading about the dangers of genetically modified foods and grain-fed meat. Or we cannot. It is absolutely MORE THAN OKAY to do the best you can with what you have. Let me just be honest here, I have been feeding my family of five on a fairly low income for a while now. I feel passionately that feeding my family a *mostly* Paleo diet is the best way to nourish all of us. I also believe that far too much pressure is put on individuals to live and eat perfectly. People are often intimidated by the potential cost of living this lifestyle that they use money as their excuse.

Money is no longer a valid excuse not to try. I rarely buy organic produce. I almost never buy grass-fed beef or wild salmon. I often eat packaged lunch meat as part of my diet and include red potatoes in recipes because I know they will fill my children up. How I am able to maintain a Paleo lifestyle may not be the best way, but it works for my family. I have still enjoyed incredible benefits from my version of this lifestyle and you can too. My recipes are all budget friendly. Later I will discuss how to reduce the financial impact of this lifestyle change. Do not pressure yourself to do more than you can. You are here, reading this book. You have taken the first step towards learning to drastically improve your life. Do the best you can because you deserve this.

Let's get started.

4. **Eat a Rainbow**

This journey does not have to be bland, boring, or a punishment for previously eating an unhealthy diet. This is your opportunity to explore the glorious foods that the earth has provided for us. Eat a variety of fruits and vegetables. Eat vibrant and beautifully colorful foods. Try fruits and vegetables you have never tried. Enjoy your personal process; fall in love with the lifestyle. Visit farmers markets that you have never been to. Try to grow something, even if it is just an herb plant or two. Feel the earth run through your fingers. Experiment with new recipes and new ingredients. Make this lifestyle enjoyable. Have fun. Life is too short not to.

5. **Get Outside**

Exercise is important. We all know that, don't we? Well I have to admit that I have never been much of an athlete. I don't exercise every single day, even though, I know I should. I find more empowerment and positive results in doing the things that I love to stay active. Earlier you read about the night I ran down dirt roads aside hay fields. I do not go to a gym. I choose to exercise in nature, and by incorporating the great outdoors into my lifestyle; I find peace and serenity that I have spent years longing for. If you love the gym, GO THERE! If you like to walk around a park, do that. If you like to hike, hike. Whatever you love, do that. Do it actively. Engage your entire mind, body, and spirit into whatever you find brings you closer to Felicity.

To Nourish

Let's talk a little more about what you ARE going to eat. Properly nutrition will transform your body and mind, building the best version of you. You already know that you will be eliminating grains, sugar, legumes, and soy. You know that you will be eating meat, vegetables, fruit, nuts, and natural sources of fat. Let's take a closer look at these nutrient rich foods and what they will do for your body, as you learn to build your own meals.

- **Protein**

  Eating a diet high in protein is essential for weight loss. Protein improves your metabolism, making your body become a fat burning machine. Your body will use the protein you feed it for energy, while building lean muscle. With a high protein diet, you will experience more satisfaction and a decrease in unhealthy cravings.

  While nuts, seeds, and some produce contain protein, your main source of protein will be the meat and eggs that you eat.

- **Carbohydrates**

  When people hear the word "carbohydrate," they immediately think of grains. Grains are incredibly high in carbohydrates. I stated earlier that a Paleo diet is typically low in carbohydrates, but you will be eating a carbohydrate with every meal. What many people don't realize is that nutrient-rich vegetables are nature's purest form of carbohydrate.

  You will be eating vegetables with every meal as your main source of carbohydrates. Fruits and most nuts are also high in carbohydrates. This is why you will be eating less of those foods. While our bodies need carbohydrates for energy, you will be limiting your carbohydrate intake so your body will burn fat for energy. You will notice quickly that fat seems to be melting off your body. You will have more energy because your body will not have to work so hard to burn through the carbohydrate-rich grains it is used to having to fight to process.

- **Fat**

  Your diet will be high in fat because - -are you ready for this? *FAT DOESN'T ACTUALLY MAKE YOU FAT!* Natural sources of fat actually provide mental clarity and extra energy. When you feed your body natural sources of fat, you are actually telling it to burn fat for energy instead of carbohydrates. This will prompt your body to use your unwanted fat stores for energy, allowing you to lose pounds effortlessly. *Your main sources of natural fats will come from avocados, nuts, seeds, oils (olive and coconut), and fatty cuts of meat.*

Earlier I said I do eat some dairy. I need to clarify: dairy is not ideal when living a Paleo lifestyle, but using clean dairy products are better than going off track completely and consuming grains. If you can go off dairy completely without struggling, that is what I recommend. I do not recommend that you eat dairy every day. I try not to have more than one serving of dairy every two days. The dairy that I occasionally consume is Greek yogurt, whey protein powder, sour cream, unsalted butter, and small servings of cheese. If you are going to choose dairy products, MAKE SURE to read labels. You want the product that is lowest in carbs and sugar. NEVER buy anything that says "Low Fat," "Reduced Fat," or "Fat Free" on the label. Remember, we want fat.

Embrace What's Real

Let's put all this information into perspective and talk about what your plate is going to look like.

☐ When planning your meals, begin by choosing your vegetable base. 1/3 to 1/2 of your plate should be covered with vegetables.

☐ Add a source of protein. Protein should make up another 1/3 of your plate.

☐ Then add a small portion of additional fat (in addition to the fat that you will get from meat).

☐ Pour a TALL glass of water to have with every meal.

☐ *With breakfast and lunch, you can add a serving of fruit if you would like. I recommend that you not eat fruit with dinner unless you are going to be working out before bed. You will not need the energy from the added carbs if you are just going to sleep.*

I will give you my favorite dinner as an example. Half my plate is covered in a heaping pile of garlic roasted asparagus and brussels sprouts (with olive oil), the other half is covered with a thick, fatty beef steak fried with coconut oil. The trick is to keep it simple. The additional fat source in this meal comes from the olive oil and coconut oil used to prepare my protein and vegetables. You are not limiting yourself or allowing your body to feel hungry. The goal is to fill up on REAL food.

Voyage: Preparedness
London Solomon

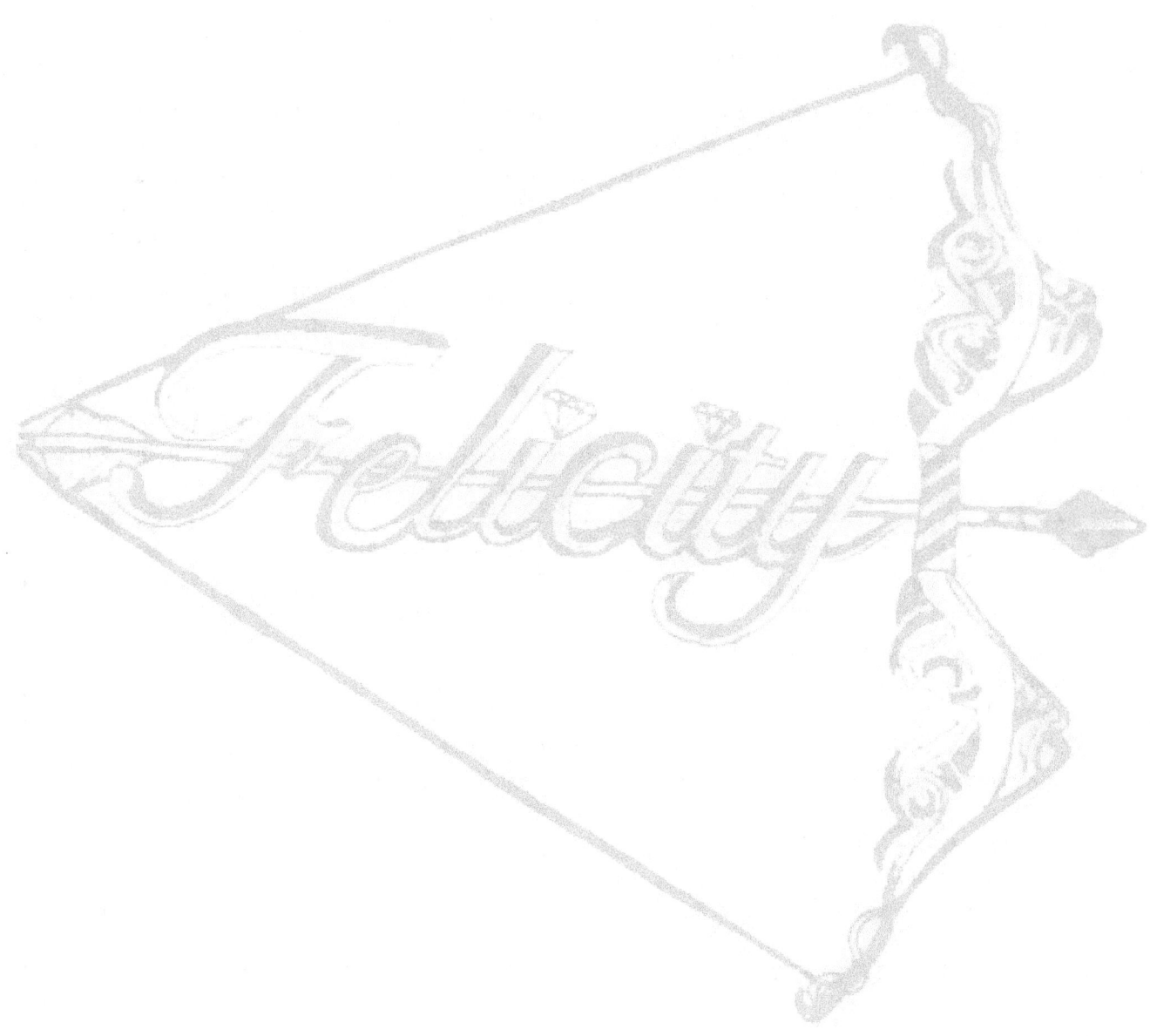

'Luck Favors the Prepared'

Preparation, planning, and commitment are KEY to successfully living a Paleo lifestyle. If you spend an extra hour or two in the kitchen every week preparing food for the meals you've planned for yourself, it is almost impossible to fail. At first, these tasks may seem tedious and like a lot of extra work, but soon you will find that your life feels more organized, productive, and staying on course will be easy. Once you begin to see results, you will be excited to plan, prepare, and eat your next week's meals. Your goal should be to only HAVE to go to the grocery store once a week.

Before you even attempt to go to the grocery store, you need to make sure that you're ready. You MUST clean out your kitchen. Ideally, you would throw out all food products that are not REAL, Paleo foods. I understand that it is difficult to throw out all non-Paleo foods when you live with others that are not ready to go Paleo with you. At the very least, throw out what will tempt you most and clear a designated section in your pantry, cupboards, refrigerator, and freezer for your food. Clean your kitchen. Wash out your refrigerator and freezer. Organize your drawers and cupboard. Create a calm atmosphere to bring your groceries home to. You kitchen is going to become your sanctuary. Make sure it is somewhere you will feel confident, rather than chaotic and overwhelmed.

Aside from groceries, there are a few items that you must have in your kitchen. Some of these you can do without, but I highly recommend you invest in the kitchen tools and supplies that will make your life easier. The cleaning supplies are a MUST, as you will be working with a lot of raw food on the same surface.

- Antibacterial surface cleaner and paper towels (or Clorox wipes)
- Antibacterial hand soap
- Latex or vinyl gloves (optional) for handling raw meat
- Water bottles!
- TUPPERWARE!
  Food storage containers with airtight lids.
  All different sizes (you'll be obsessed with these containers soon, trust me).
- Gallon, quart, and sandwich sized Ziploc bags
- A black sharpie (for writing on bags)
- Aluminum foil
- Parchment paper
- Sharp kitchen knife set
- 2 cutting boards (one for fruits and vegetables, one for meat)
- Medium sauce pan
- Large skillet

- Large stainless steel pot
- 2 cup glass measuring cup
- Measurement spoon set
- Wooden spoon
- "Potato" masher
- Metal spatula
- Kitchen timer
- Large baking dish
- Vegetable peeler
- Large mixing bowl

Highly Recommended Appliances:

- *Blender*
- *Large food processor*
- *Coffee pot (for coffee and tea)*
- *Juicer (there are no juicing recipes in this book but, eventually, you will want a juicer)*

Now that your kitchen is ready, you can start thinking about your first meal plan. After you read this entire book, meal planning will be simple. Don't get overwhelmed! Remember that you bought this book for a reason and, and that at the end, I have provided easy worksheets to guide you through this process. You are going to plan one week's worth of meals at a time. For now, I will give you an example of one day's plan. Be sure to incorporate these "rules" with all meals. Snacks should be small and only if you feel that you need them. Also, I have to admit that I do not always eat a vegetable with breakfast. It is very important to eat breakfast, as it sets your metabolism's pace for the day, but if you have a hard time with breakfast (like I do) just be sure that you start your day with protein and fat.

	Monday
Water	[ ] 20 oz. [ ] 20 oz. [ ] 20 oz. [ ] 20 oz. [ ] 20 oz. [ ] 20 oz.
Breakfast	*2 fried eggs, 2 strips of bacon, 1 cup strawberries*
Snack	*Cucumber slices*
Lunch	*Turkey wrap with cashews*
Snack	*Apple*
Dinner	*Avocado double burger with sweet potato fries*
Exercise?	*Walked 1 mile at 7 pm*

You will make a meal plan, like the one above, for every day of the week. In the beginning; you will need to check the recipes you plan to use, write down all ingredients used (with measurements), and then check your kitchen to cross off any ingredients you already have. Do not make your shopping list until you have done this for every recipe for the entire week.

A few things to consider while planning your meals and grocery lists:

- *Plan your grocery trips on a day that you will have time to spend in the kitchen, as soon as you get home from the grocery store, preparing the food you just bought. It is too easy to put off meal prep if you don't do it before the food is even put away. Don't set yourself up for failure. Expect to spend at least an hour in the kitchen when you get home from the store.*
- *Find out what meat is on sale. If you find a good deal on meat or produce, save yourself some money and incorporate sale items in the next week's meal plan.*
- *Go big! When shopping for meat, always buy larger packages (or in bulk) when you can. When cooking large quantities of meat, refrigerate what you think you and your family will eat over the next 3 days and freeze the rest. It can always be used later and you don't want to eat the same thing every day all week.*
- *Take a look at your work or other schedules. Plan meals appropriately around work and other events.*
- *Plan on making extra dinner every night to save and eat for lunch the next day. This will save you time and money.*
- *Keep it simple. This doesn't have to be extravagant. Have fun with some days' meals but don't plan to make a 5 course meal every night.*

- *Don't forget snacks!*
- *Try one new item every week.*
- *When making your grocery list, keep in mind the needs/wants of others in your home. If you live and shop for people who are not ready to go Paleo, be sure to add their items to your list so you don't have to go back to the store.*

Do not write a grocery list until you have filled in your meal plan for the entire next week and written down the amount of each ingredient you need for each recipe, then you can look over your recipes and compile common ingredients. If you write "*1/2 white onion*" on your grocery list four times for four different recipes you will end up with an overwhelming list. You will need 2 white onions. Simplify. Now that you have your grocery list, grab your meal plan and shopping list and head to the store! Stick to your list. Don't make last minute alterations unless you absolutely have to.

Honey I'm Home

When you get home from the store, place all your produce (except berries) in a clean sink full of cold water to wash them. Take a look at the snacks you've planned for the week and prepare all of them. They should be fairly simple. Store your snacks in Ziploc bags or Tupperware. Cut up all your produce the day you buy it. Even if you aren't planning to pre-cook every meal, make sure the produce is ready when you are. This will make you less likely to change your menu or make excuses for not preparing the planned meal later. If any of the meat you plan on eating can be pre-cooked, cook it now. Make sure to let it cool before placing it in closed Tupperware containers. Label all Ziploc bags and Tupperware containers with contents and date prepared. You can also write the day you plan on eating the item on them to help keep yourself organized. If you are planning to have a crockpot meal, put all ingredients to the recipe in a gallon sized bag to freeze. When you're ready to put your meal in the crockpot, you just have to pour everything out of the bag.

You can pre-cook all your meals if you feel that it will help you be most successful. People that have very little time during the week find this most beneficial. Personally, I enjoy cooking a few times a week so I just prepare the ingredients and precook meals for the days I know I won't have the extra time. Whatever works best for you.

> *Sanitize your prep area and cutting boards and wash your hands in between each item prepared to avoid cross contamination.*

Voyage: Cookbook
London Solomon

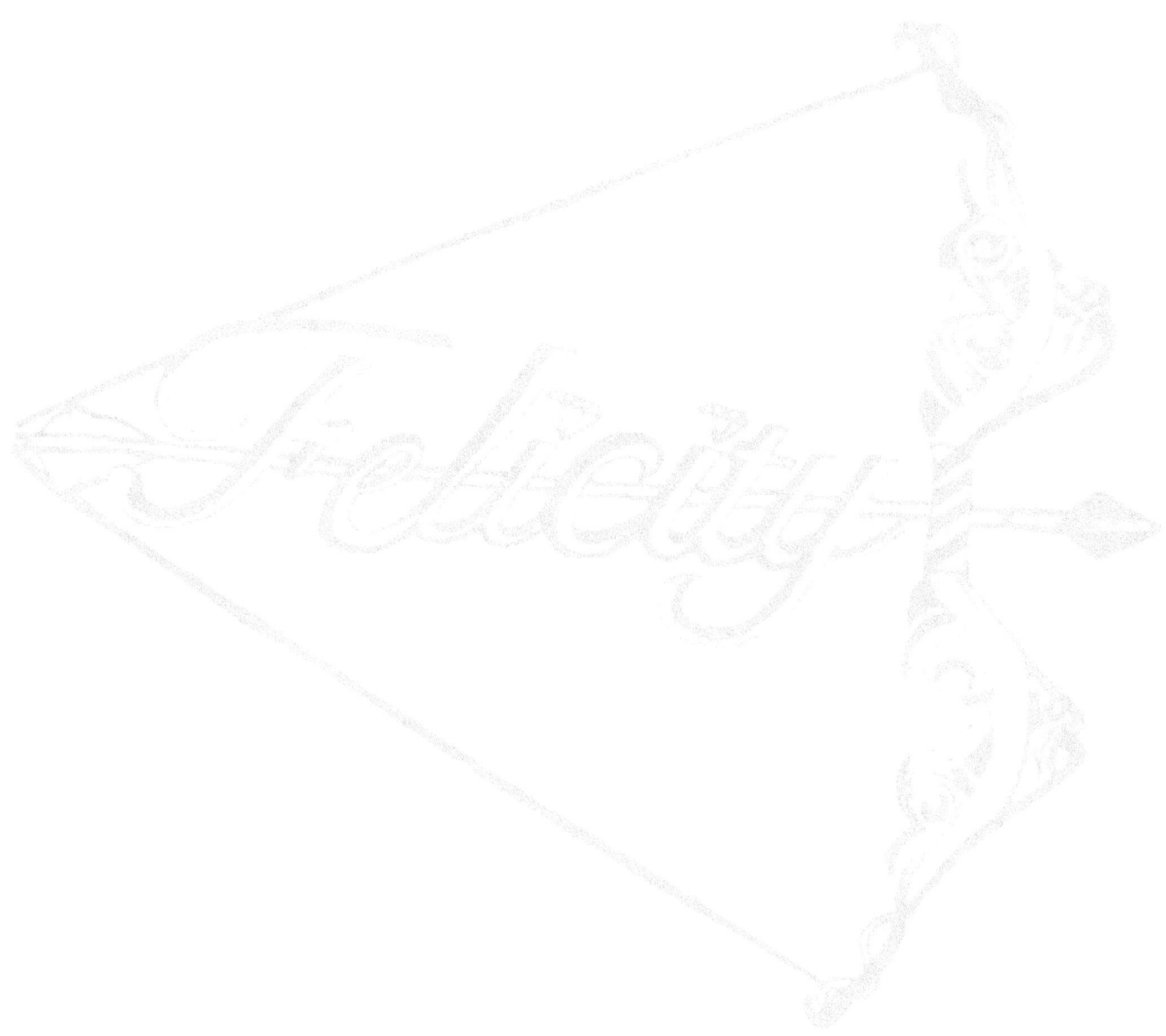

Rise and Shine

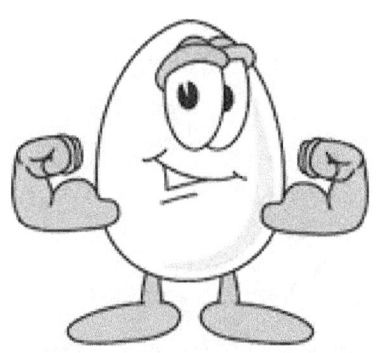

Breakfast REALLY is the most important meal of the day! Make sure to start your day off with WATER, protein, and fat. If you are going to have a busy, active day get some healthy carbs in too. Fruit is always an easy way to get your healthy carbs in first thing in the morning, but if you don't want to feel hungry and irritable in a few hours, eat your eggs or some meat! Eggs and meat can be pre-cooked and refrigerated for those of you who hate mornings as much as I do. Make it work, it will be worth it!

Eggs

Scramble 'em, fry 'em, poach 'em, or have them hard boiled. However you like your eggs, do that! Eggs are an excellent source of protein and will keep you full and mentally focused throughout your mornings. Use olive oil or coconut oil to grease your pans and add a little extra healthy fat to your breakfast. Have a little extra time? Try my *Cowboy Omelet*!

Cowboy Omelet

This hearty recipe will leave you ready to tackle your day,
keeping you energized and satisfied for hours!

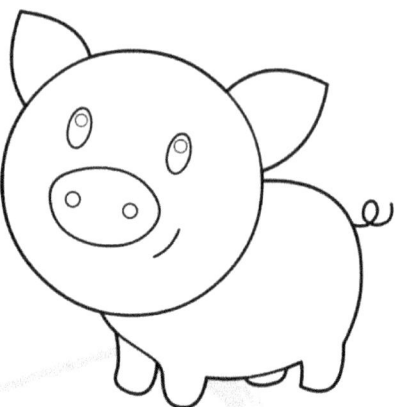

Ingredients:
- 3 eggs
- 2 TBSP water
- ½ tsp paprika
- 1 tsp dried parsley
- Salt and Pepper (to taste)
- A dash of cayenne pepper (if you like a little extra kick)
- ¼ cup browned ground sausage
- ¼ cup diced ham
- 1 TBSP finely chopped onion
- Peppers of choice
  (use finely chopped fresh peppers or canned green chilies, whatever you prefer)
- Olive Oil for frying pan

Directions:
1. Prepare whatever combination of ingredients you've chosen to use as the filling of your scrumptious omelet. Brown your sausage, dice your ham, chop your onion, and prepare your peppers. Mix it all together in a small mixing bowl and add a little seasoning salt, if you'd like. Set the mixture aside.
2. In a medium mixing bowl; use a whisk to beat eggs, water, paprika, parsley, cayenne pepper, salt, and pepper until frothy. Drizzle olive oil in your pan and pre-heat medium frying pan on the stove at medium heat.
3. Slowly pour egg mixture into your frying pan. If you have a lid, place it over the pan for 1-2 minutes.
4. Place your prepared filling in the center of your omelet. Using a spatula, careful fold half of the omelet over and allow it to cook on one side for 30 seconds to a minute. Then, carefully flip the omelet over and finish cooking it on the other side.
5. When the omelet is cooked thoroughly, slide it onto a plate, let cool, and enjoy!

Shake It Up!

Because who has time for eggs every day?

If you are not a morning eater and just want something quick and easy that you can drink on your way out the door, consider a protein packed smoothie. You can use liquid egg whites (if you are trying to stay strictly paleo) or whey protein powder in your smoothies, whichever you prefer. Try to throw in a few veggies and make all your smoothies green. This is an excellent way to start your day, fueling your body with protein and nutritious produce.

The Chocolate Monkey
Makes 1 smoothie.

Ingredients:
- 1 banana; sliced and frozen (slice up a few on pre-day to have in the freezer to add a delicious, creamy texture to your smoothies)
- 1-2 scoop of chocolate whey protein OR ½ cup of liquid egg whites and 2 TBS cocoa powder
- 2 TBSP peanut or almond butter (you may also use PB2, which is powdered peanut butter. I highly recommend it!)
- ½ an avocado
- 1 cup almond or coconut milk
- ½ cup ice

Throw all your ingredients in a blender and BLEND!

Razzle-Dazzle Island Life
Makes 1 smoothie

Ingredients:
- ½ banana; sliced and frozen
- ¼ cup raspberries (frozen or fresh)
- ½ cup cubed pineapple or mango (fresh or frozen)
- 1 tsp chai seeds
- 1-2 scoops scoop vanilla whey protein or 1 cup liquid egg whites
- 1 handful fresh spinach
- 1 ½ cup almond milk
- Add ice as desired

Throw all your ingredients in a blender and BLEND!

Avo-Heaven
4 servings

Ingredients:

- 2 large avocados
- 3 eggs
- 1 slice cooked bacon, chopped into bits
- ½ tsp paprika
- ½ tsp garlic salt
- 1 tsp finely chopped green onion
- 1 tsp finely chopped fresh parsley
- Sea salt and pepper to taste

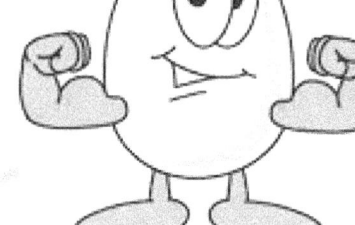

Directions:

1. Preheat oven to 425 degrees
2. Slice avocados in half and remove the pits. Scoop a little more of the avocado out, forming a pit or "bowl" in which you will later pour your egg mixture.
3. In a medium mixing bowl; whisk together the eggs, bacon bits, paprika, garlic salt, sea salt, and pepper.
4. Place your avocado halves on a cookie sheet with the open pit facing upwards. Using a small measuring cup, carefully pour your egg mixture into the avocados. Do not fill them all the way up because the egg will rise as it bakes.
5. Sprinkle the chopped onion and parsley over the top of your avocados and carefully place the cookie sheet in your preheated oven. Bake for 15 minutes or until the egg is fully cooked.
6. After removing your Avo-Eggs from the oven, feel free to add toppings if you desire. I like to add a little shredding cheese and sometimes a drop of sour cream. Don't be afraid to play with this recipe and make it your own!

Sweet Treat Acorn Squash

Ingredients:
- 1 acorn squash
- 2 TBSP honey
- 3 TBSP coconut oil, melted
- 2 TBSP sugar free maple syrup
- 1-2 tsp ground cinnamon

Directions:
1. Preheat oven to 350 degrees.
2. Cut squash in half lengthwise and scrape out seeds.
3. Place both halves, meat down, on an oiled cookie sheet.
4. Bake for 20 minutes.
5. While squash is baking, prepare your glaze by stirring honey, melted coconut oil, and syrup together in a small mixing bowl.
6. Carefully turn both halves of the squash over so you can see the meat of the squash. Leave on cookie sheet.
7. Brush honey glaze all over meat of the squash. Poor excess glaze into the bowl of each squash half.
8. Sprinkle desired amount of cinnamon on top of squash halves.
9. Return the cookie sheet to the oven for an additional 20 minutes.
10. Cool until you can handle.
11. You can eat this deliciously sweet treat with a spoon or fork, straight out of the rind. Enjoy!

The Seuss Casserole
12 servings

Ingredients:
- 10 eggs
- 1 avocado; sliced in half, cut into cubes, and spoon out of the shell
- ½ cup diced ham
- 1 cup ground pork sausage (browned)
- 2 cups shredded zucchini (it is easiest to shred zucchini in a food processor but you can also do it manually, using a cheese grater)
- ½ chopped green bell peppers
- Sea salt and pepper to taste
- 2/3 cup shredded cheddar cheese (optional)

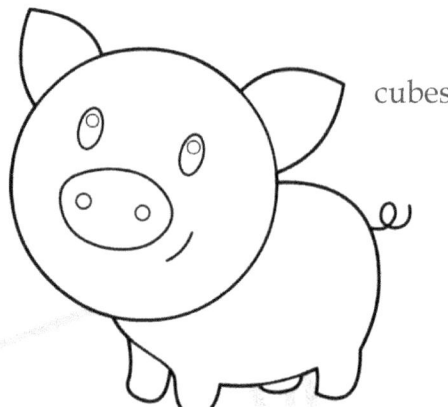 cubes

Directions:
1. Preheat oven to 375 degrees.
2. In a medium mixing bowl combine avocado cubes, diced ham, ground sausage, and chopped bell peppers and set aside.
3. In a large mixing bowl whisk all 10 eggs. Next, stir the zucchini, salt, and pepper into the eggs. Then stir the meat mixture in with the eggs and zucchini.
4. Use olive oil or coconut oil to grease a large baking or casserole pan (ceramic or glass work best). Pour the combined ingredients from the large mixing bowl into the casserole pan and cover with tin foil.
5. Bake covered casserole for 40-50 minutes.
6. Take your casserole out of the oven and remove the tinfoil. If you would like to add cheese, sprinkle the shredded cheese over the top of the casserole now. If not, just remove the tin foil. Place the casserole in the oven and bake an additional 10 minutes.

Cinnamon Flap Jacks
8 servings

Ingredients:
- 2 cups almond flour
- 4 eggs
- 1 cup small curd cottage cheese
- 2 tsp baking powder
- 1 TBSP cinnamon
- ½ cup coconut milk
- 3 TBSP honey (or stevia)

Directions:
1. Combine almond flour, eggs, cottage cheese, and baking powder in a large mixing bowl. Using an electric mixer, mix ingredients on a high speed for about 30 seconds.
2. Stir in cinnamon, coconut milk, and honey or stevia.
3. Preheat a large frying pan and use butter, olive oil, or coconut oil to grease the pan.
4. Poor ¼ cup to ½ cup of the pancake batter into the frying pan. When you see the sides of your pancake browning and bubbles forming in the uncooked batter, flip pancake over. This should only take 1-2 minutes on each side.
5. Repeat until you've used up all your batter.
6. You may use sugar free syrup on your pancakes or make your own cinnamon syrup (recipe below).

Cinnamon Syrup
- 2 TBS melted butter
- 1 TBS melted coconut oil
- 2 tsp cinnamon
- ¼ cup honey

Life is Too Short For Boring Salads

While starting your day out strong with a protein-packed breakfast, you must give just as much attention to the rest of the meals you feed your body throughout the day. Salads are always an easy option for packed lunches. You can throw just about any combination of meat and vegetables together and form an easy, healthy lunch. Be adventurous with salads and take a little time on your meal prep day to experiment with different ideas.

Carne Asada Taco Salad

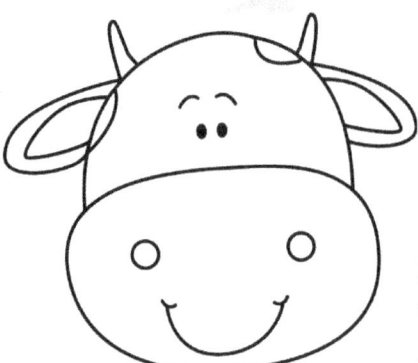

Ingredients:
- 3 pounds flank steak
- 1 medium red onion
- ½ cup fresh cilantro
- ½ cup balsamic vinegar
- ¼ cup olive oil
- ¼ cup beef broth
- ¼ cup soy sauce
- 1 (15-ounce) can diced tomatoes
- 1 (4-ounce) can diced green chilies
- 3 limes
- ¼ cup chili powder OR 2 packets of preferred taco seasoning packet
- 1 tsp paprika
- 2 tsp oregano
- 2 teaspoons cumin
- 1 clove of garlic, minced (approximately 2 tablespoons)
- 2 TBSP black pepper
- 1 tsp sea salt

Directions:

1. Finely chop onion, cilantro, and garlic. Place chopped ingredients in a large mixing bowl.

2. Slice all 3 limes into 4 wedges each. Squeeze the juice out of all but 2 of the wedges into the bowl with the other produce. Disregard the wedges that were juiced and place the remaining 2 wedges in the bowl.

3. Add the diced tomatoes, green chilies, balsamic vinegar, olive oil, beef broth, and soy sauce into the bowl. Stir all the ingredients together.

4. Add chili powder (or taco seasoning), paprika, oregano, cumin, black pepper, and salt to the marinade mixture. Stir spices into the marinade.

5. Add beef into the marinade. You can, then, poor the marinating meat into a gallon sized bag or cover the bowl and stick it in the refrigerator to marinate.

6. Allow meat to marinate for at least 4 hours (*see quick tips for ideal marinating times and methods*).

7. Once you are ready to cook your carne asada, poor the meat and marinade through a strainer over your sink. Pull the beef out of the colander and place it on another plate. Leave the remaining vegetables in the colander.

8. Slowly fry your beef strips on the stove with 2 tablespoons of olive oil at a low-medium heat until they are browned (or as thoroughly cooked as you prefer).

9. While your beef is frying, prepare your salad.

10. Remove the cooked meat from the frying pan. While the meat cools, sauté the leftover vegetables from the marinade in the olive oil and beef juices left in the frying pan for 2-3 minutes.

11. Mix Carne Asada beef, sautéed vegetables, and whatever other topping of your choice to your salad.

12. ENJOY!

Quick Tips:

☐ I prefer to make the marinade the night before I intend to make this recipe, so the beef has been soaking in this deliciousness all night. The vinegar tenderizes the beef and the other flavorful ingredients soak in to the meat.

☐ My other favorite way to prepare this recipe is to prepare the marinade, add the beef, and then throw it in the freezer to use another night (awesome freezer meal to put together on prep-day).

☐ If you don't make the marinade the day (or days) before the night you wish to enjoy this recipe, it will still be delicious if only marinated for a few hours. Keep in the fridge until you're ready to get cookin'.

☐ Sometimes it is less expensive to purchase a large beef roast and cut it up to use as flank steak (used in this recipe), stew meat, etc.

☐ Bottled minced garlic isn't as strongly flavored as freshly minced garlic is, but it's a big timesaver and still offers the same garlic flavor. When using bottled garlic for this recipe, use 3 tablespoons.

Bailar en La Boca Salad

"Dance in Your Mouth" Crockpot Taco Salad

Ingredients:

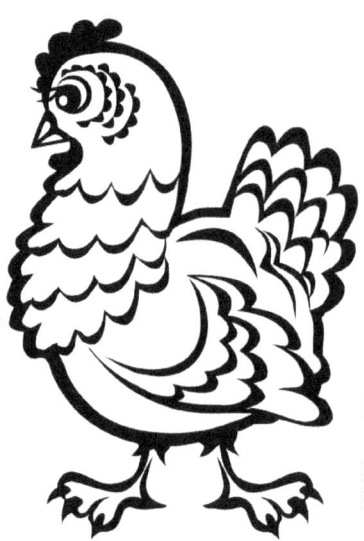

- 3-4 lbs boneless, skinless chicken breasts
- 2 cans diced tomatoes
- 1 small can tomato sauce
- 2 small cans diced chili peppers
- 1 small can diced jalapeños (optional)
- 1 cup chicken broth
- 1 white onion, chopped
- 2 taco seasoning packets
- 1 ranch seasoning packet

Directions:

1. Set thawed chicken breasts in large crock pot.
2. In a small mixing bowl combine canned tomatoes, tomato sauce, peppers, chicken broth, and chopped onion. Stir seasoning packets into sauce mixture.
3. Pour the ingredients from your mixing bowl over the chicken breasts in the crockpot.
4. Allow chicken to cook in your crockpot, on low, for 4-6 hours or until it is falling apart.
5. When the chicken is falling apart, pull it out of the crockpot and shred it. It should just pull apart.
6. Place shredded chicken in a bowl or storage container and dish desired amount of tomato sauce over the chicken.
7. Serve over green, leafy vegetables of your choice. Feel free to add peppers or whatever other vegetables you'd like. The sauce makes an excellent dressing! Add full fat sour cream, avocado, and/or a little shredded cheese if you'd like.
8. Refrigerate leftovers in individual portions for easy lunches.

Sweetheart's Chicken Salad

Ingredients:

- 3 lbs boneless, skinless chicken breasts
- 2 tsp garlic salt
- 3 TBSP ranch seasoning powder
- 1 small white onion; finely minced
- 2 TBSP minced garlic
- ¼ cup balsamic vinegar
- ½ cup honey
- 1 lemon's juice (cut in half and squeeze by hand)
- 1 tsp lemon zest
- 2 TBSP olive oil
- 2 tsp red wine vinegar
- Season salt
- Salt and pepper

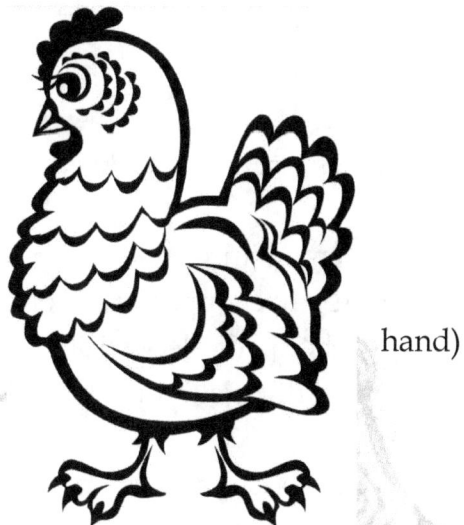

Directions:

1. Preheat oven to 425 degrees.
2. Place chicken breasts on greased cookie sheet.
3. Sprinkle seasoning salt and pepper over chicken and bake for 20 minutes or until they are cooked all the way through.
4. While the chicken is baking; put all remaining ingredients listed above in a blender to make a delightful, sweet dressing.
5. When the chicken breasts are fully cooked, allow them to cool, and slice them into ½" thick strips. Place strips in a gallon sized Ziploc bag.
6. Poor approximately 2/3 of your dressing over the chicken, in the Ziploc bag.
7. Poor the remaining dressing in a mason jar and refrigerate.
8. Allow the chicken to marinate overnight in the dressing.
9. Later, divide the chicken into individual servings. Add desired amount of additional dressing to individual portions.
10. Serve over green, leafy vegetables of your choice. Feel free to add peppers or whatever other vegetables you'd like. Olives and yellow peppers go fabulously with this recipe!

Here Fishy-Fishy!
Canned Tuna or Salmon Wrap

Ingredients:
- 1 avocado
- 2 (5 oz) cans tuna or salmon (in water)
- 2 TBSP lemon juice
- 1 TBSP finely chopped green onion
- 1 finely chopped celery stick
- 1 chopped dill pickle or 2 TBS. dill relish
- 2 tsp finely chopped fresh parsley
- Salt and lemon pepper to taste

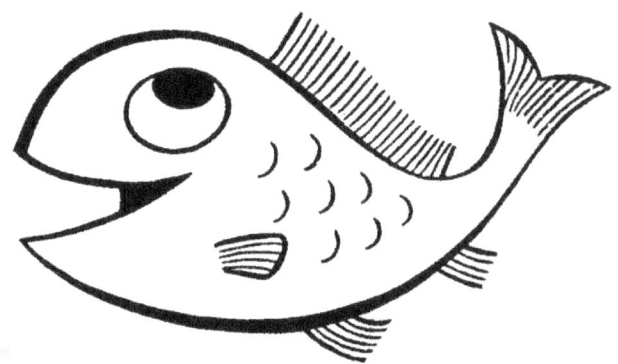

Directions:
1. Open the cans of fish and drain the water out of them. Spoon fish into a medium sized mixing bowl.
2. Add lemon juice, onion, celery, and pickle or relish in to your mixing bowl.
3. Using a rubber spatula, mix ingredients together. Make sure to scrape the side of the bowl as you stir it all together.
4. Cut avocado in half, remove pit. Carefully cut into the avocado horizontally and vertically forming cube-like chunks, being sure not to pierce the shell (do this to both halves).
   -for a creamier texture, make avocado chunks smaller so they blend into the tuna mixture
5. Scoop the avocado chunks into your fish mixture.
6. Add parsley, salt, and lemon pepper to your bowl and mix it all together.

You can eat this fish salad however you like (using Paleo foods). A few of my favorite ways to prepare it are;
- ☐ Over a green salad with a combination of spinach, cabbage, and iceberg lettuce
- ☐ As a wrap, in a large romaine lettuce leaf
- ☐ With sliced cucumbers, as a dip or spooned on lop of cucumber slices

When You Fail to Prepare, You Prepare to Fail

Crockpot and Freezer Meals to Assemble on Meal Prep Day

Taking the time to prepare freezer and crockpot meals is one of the best ways to reduce stress, save time later, and set yourself up for success on even the busiest days. The recipes in this section are my family's absolute favorite freezer meals so keep in mind that they are portioned to accommodate 5 people. They can be doubled for larger families or extra meals. They can also be cut in half for smaller portions, but I would recommend making a larger portion and splitting it into 2 bags for extra meals.

One concern I hear ALL THE TIME from single people is that they have a hard time preparing meals for only one person. If this is your situation; prepare these recipes and divide them into quart sized bags (rather than gallon bags). I also recommend that, when preparing crockpot meals, you prepare 2 portions because there's nothing better than an easy dinner and delicious leftovers for lunch the next day.

Let's Get Down to Business

Below is a list of the recipes that will be in this section.
They are, by no means, the only recipes in the book that you can prepare and freeze.

1. **Meatloaf**

2. **Kickin' Cranberry Chicken**

3. **Hearty Beef Stew**

4. **White Chicken Chili**

5. **Apple Pork Tenderloin**

6. **Turkey Breast**

- *A little tip to save you some cash:* You can buy carne asada and beef stew meat at most grocery stores, but I always find it much cheaper to buy a small roast and cut it up myself. Totally up to you though.
- *And a little tip to save time:* Rather than buying garlic cloves and chopping them up myself, I buy minced garlic in a bottle. We use lots of garlic and it's super convenient!

Before we get to the recipes, let's first talk about how we're going to stay organized and efficient while preparing several different meals in the same area. Take note of the items you will need to have, in addition to ingredients, to prepare your meals successfully.

o   It is very important that you make sure to clean your workspace with an **antibacterial soap** and **a clean rag or paper towel** each time you wipe down your workspace.

o   You will need a **large workspace**. Lay all your ingredients out, separating and organizing them so they are easy to find.

o   **Gallon (and/or quart) sized freezer bags** and **a black permanent marker**. Label each of your gallon sized bags. Write which meal it contains, the method and amount of time it needs to cook (and at what temperature; low/high for crockpot or degree for oven), any ingredients (usually liquids) that need to be added, and which side dishes you'd like to have with your meal (as a reminder to prepare them).

o   You will need **2 cutting boards.** Use one for meat and the other for produce to prevent cross contamination. The meat's cutting board MUST be cleaned between each use/meat.

o   Start by chopping and preparing all the produce you will need for all recipes being prepared. Unless the recipe specifies that you steam or sauté produce in advance, measure the produce and put it in the appropriate bag.

o   Prepare all canned ingredients. Open all the cans and drain the ones that need to be. Poor the cans into their designated bags.
    Typically broths are not frozen but added at the time you prepare the recipe.
    Do not open cans of broth for the purpose of freezing unless a recipe specifically instructs you too.
    Frozen liquids take up extra freezer space and it isn't really necessary to pre-pour broth.

o   Measure and add all spices and seasonings to the appropriate bags.

o   Prepare meat as explained in the recipe and place it in its bag. It is typically better to pre-cook ground meats, especially if you plan to use a crockpot. I always brown hamburger, sausage, and any other ground meat because if you don't, it turns out mushy and a little slimy. Trust me on this one.
    Don't forget to thoroughly clean your workspace, tools, and cutting board between each use.

o   Seal the bags and gently shake and roll them around to combine all the ingredients.

o   If you have the space, it is easiest to lie all your bags flat on a cookie sheet until they are frozen. Then they are thinner and more compact than if all the ingredients were to all be frozen at the bottom of the bag. If you can't do that, don't sweat it. Just toss them in the freezer where they will fit.

o   When you want to use one of your meals, take it out of the freezer and put it in the refrigerator 1 or 2 days in advance.

Momma's Sneaky Meatloaf
They won't ever know how many veggies they're eating.
It'll be our secret.

Ingredients:

- 2 lbs ground beef
- 1 can diced tomatoes
- 1 can tomato sauce
- 3 eggs
- 1 onion soup packet
- ½ head cauliflower, shredded
- ¼ cup almond flour
- 1 tsp garlic powder
- 1 tsp minced garlic
- Season salt and pepper to taste

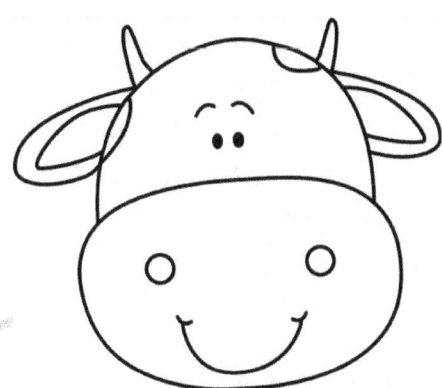

Directions:

1. Label gallon sized bag using permanent marker,
   "Paleo Meatloaf:
   +Thaw and place in bread pan
   +Cover with tinfoil and cook at 375 degrees for 50 minutes
   +Take meatloaf out of the oven after 50 minutes, remove tinfoil, and pour drippings out of pan.
   +Place meatloaf back in oven (uncovered) for an additional 20 minutes."
2. In a medium mixing bowl; mix together diced tomatoes, tomato sauce, eggs, onion soup packet, almond flour, garlic powder, minced garlic, season salt, and pepper.
3. In a large mixing bowl; stir together raw ground beef and shredded cauliflower.
4. Pour tomato mixture into large mixing bowl. Using a mixer, mix all ingredients for 1 continuous minute.
5. Spoon meatloaf into labeled gallon sized bag and freeze.

Kickin' Cranberry Chicken

Ingredients:

- 4 lbs boneless, skinless chicken breasts
- 1 cans cranberry sauce (no sugar added)
- 1 TBSP red wine vinegar
- 1 (16 oz.) bottle Catalina salad dressing
- 1 cup cranberries (fresh or frozen)
- 1 onion soup packet
- 1 ranch powder packet

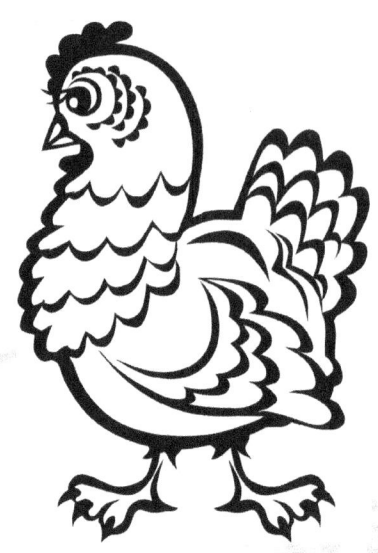

Directions:

1. Label gallon sized bag using permanent marker,
   "Kickin' Cranberry Chicken: Crockpot
   +Cook on low for 4-6 hours"
2. Place chicken breasts inside gallon sized bag.
3. Pour remaining ingredients in bag, over chicken.
4. Seal bag and mix ingredients by shaking and rolling bag. Slightly open and squeeze bag to release as much excess air as possible, flattening meal for easier storage.
5. Freeze until you're ready to use.

Hearty Beef Stew

Ingredients:

- 2-3 lbs beef stew meat
- 1 sweet potato, cut into chunks (your preference of size)
- 1 cup chopped celery
- ½-1 cup kale, chopped (your preference of size)
- ½ cup chopped carrots
- 2 zucchini, diced
- 1 medium white onion, finely chopped
- 1 TBSP finely chopped minced garlic
- 1 (14.5 oz) can petite diced tomatoes
- ¼ cup tomato paste
- ¼ cup balsamic vinegar
- 1 tsp honey
- 1 TBSP liquid smoke
- 1 tsp dried thyme
- 2 TBSP dried parsley
- 3-5 dried bay leaves
- Season salt and pepper to taste
- 2 cups beef broth
- 3 TBSP almond flour
- 2 tsp corn starch

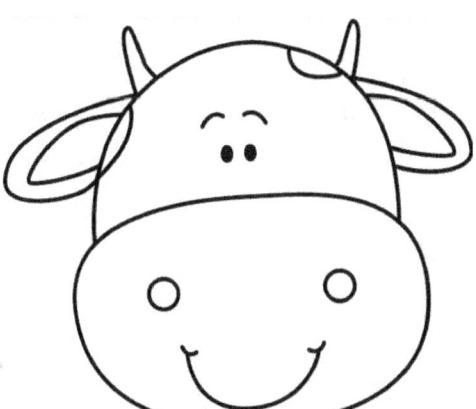

Directions:

1. 1 gallon sized bag using permanent marker,
   "Hearty Beef Stew: Crockpot
   +Add 1 cup beef broth to crockpot
   +Cook on low for 4 hours
   +Whisk 1 cup beef broth, almond flour, and cornstarch together and pour it into stew (to thicken).
   +Continue cooking on low 1 more hour"
2. Pour can of petite diced tomatoes (use all contents of can, do not strain), tomato paste, garlic, balsamic vinegar, honey, liquid smoke, thyme, parsley, bay leaves, season salt, and pepper into gallon sized bag.
3. Shake and roll bag to combine ingredients.

(Continued on Page 41)

4. Add potatoes, celery, kale, carrots, zucchini, onion, and stew meat to bag.

5. Seal bag and mix ingredients by shaking and rolling bag.

6. Slightly open and squeeze bag to release as much excess air as possible, flattening meal for easier storage.

7. Freeze until you're ready to use.

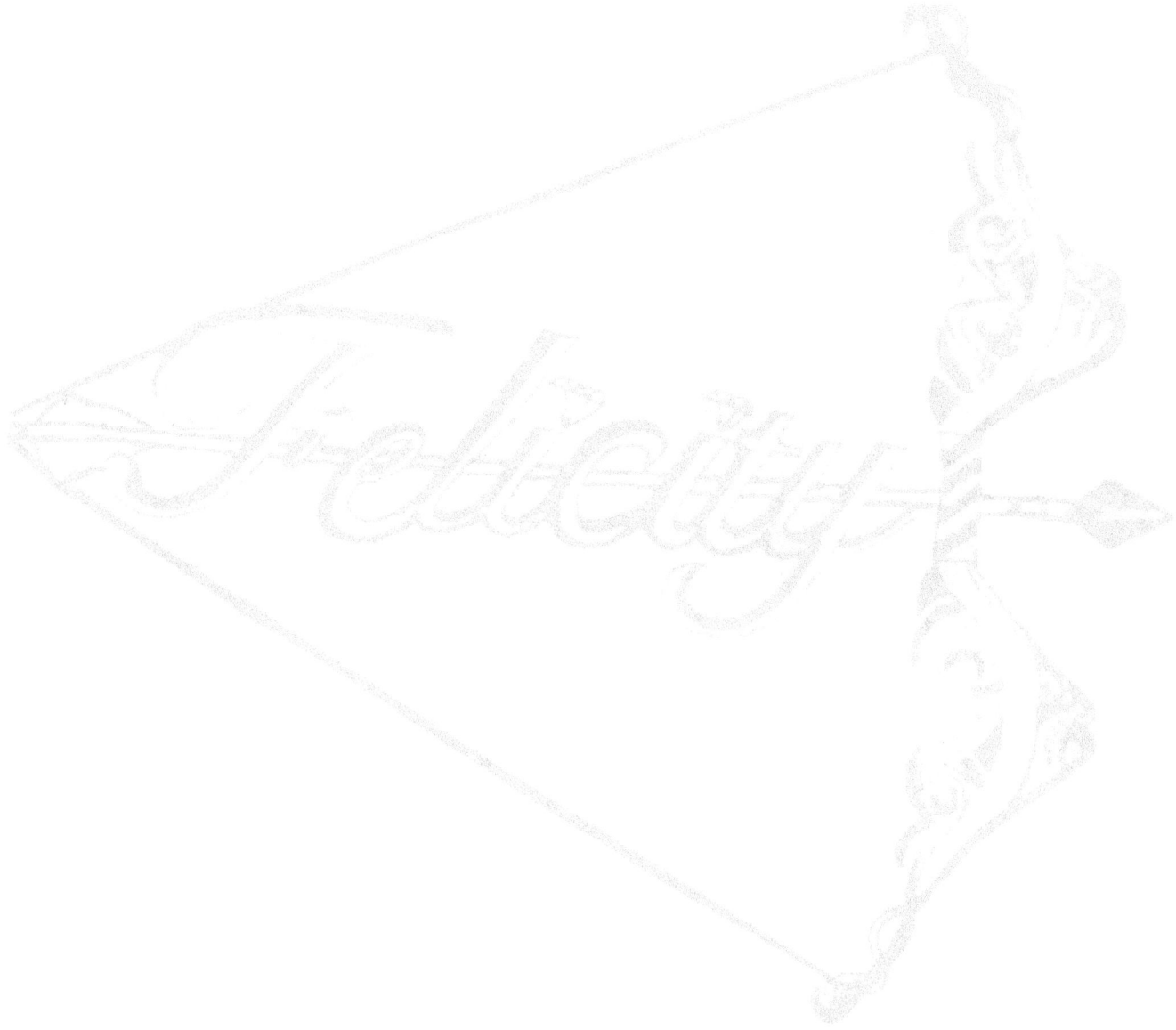

Cha-Cha-Chicken Chili

Ingredients:
- 3 (12.5 oz.) cans, fully cooked, chunk chicken in water
- 1 tsp olive oil
- 2 cups coconut milk
- 2 TBSP fresh cilantro, minced
- 1 medium yellow onion, finely chopped
- 1 (14.5 oz.) can diced tomatoes
- 3 TBSP tomato paste
- 1 (2.5 oz.) can green chilies
- 1 jalapeno, finely diced (*optional*)
- 1 green bell pepper, chopped
- ¼ cup lime juice
- 1 tsp garlic salt
- ½ tsp cayenne pepper
- 1 TBSP paprika
- 2 tsp cumin
- 3 TBSP chili powder
- Salt and pepper to taste
  Ingredient to be added to finished chili:
- 2 avocados

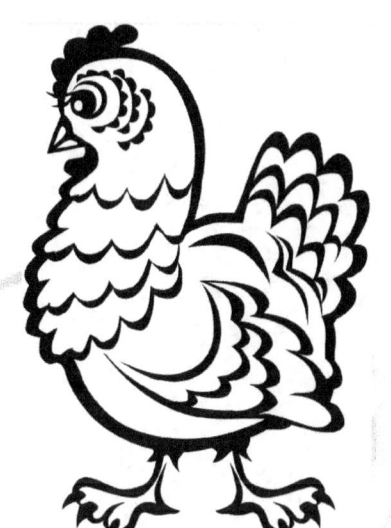

Directions:
1. Label gallon sized bag,
   "White Chicken Chili: Crockpot
   +Cook on low/med 4 hours
   +Add avocado chunks to finished chili"
2. Open cans of chicken, strain excess liquid, and pour into gallon sized bag.
3. Add cilantro, onion, all contents of diced tomatoes can, all contents of green chiles can, tomato paste, jalapeno, bell pepper, garlic salt, cayenne pepper, paprika, cumin, chili powder, salt, and pepper.
4. Shake and roll sealed bag to mix ingredients.
5. Open bag, add olive oil, coconut milk, and lime juice. Shake and roll contents, mixing all ingredients thoroughly.
6. Slightly open and squeeze bag to release as much excess air as possible, flattening meal for easier storage.

(Continued on Page 43)

7. Freeze until you're ready to use.

While chili is in crockpot, prepare avocado to add to finished recipe (as desired) by cutting avocado in half, removing the pit. Then carefully cut into the avocado horizontally and vertically forming cube-like chunks, being sure not to pierce the shell (do this to both halves).
*for a creamier texture, make avocado chunks smaller so they blend into chili.

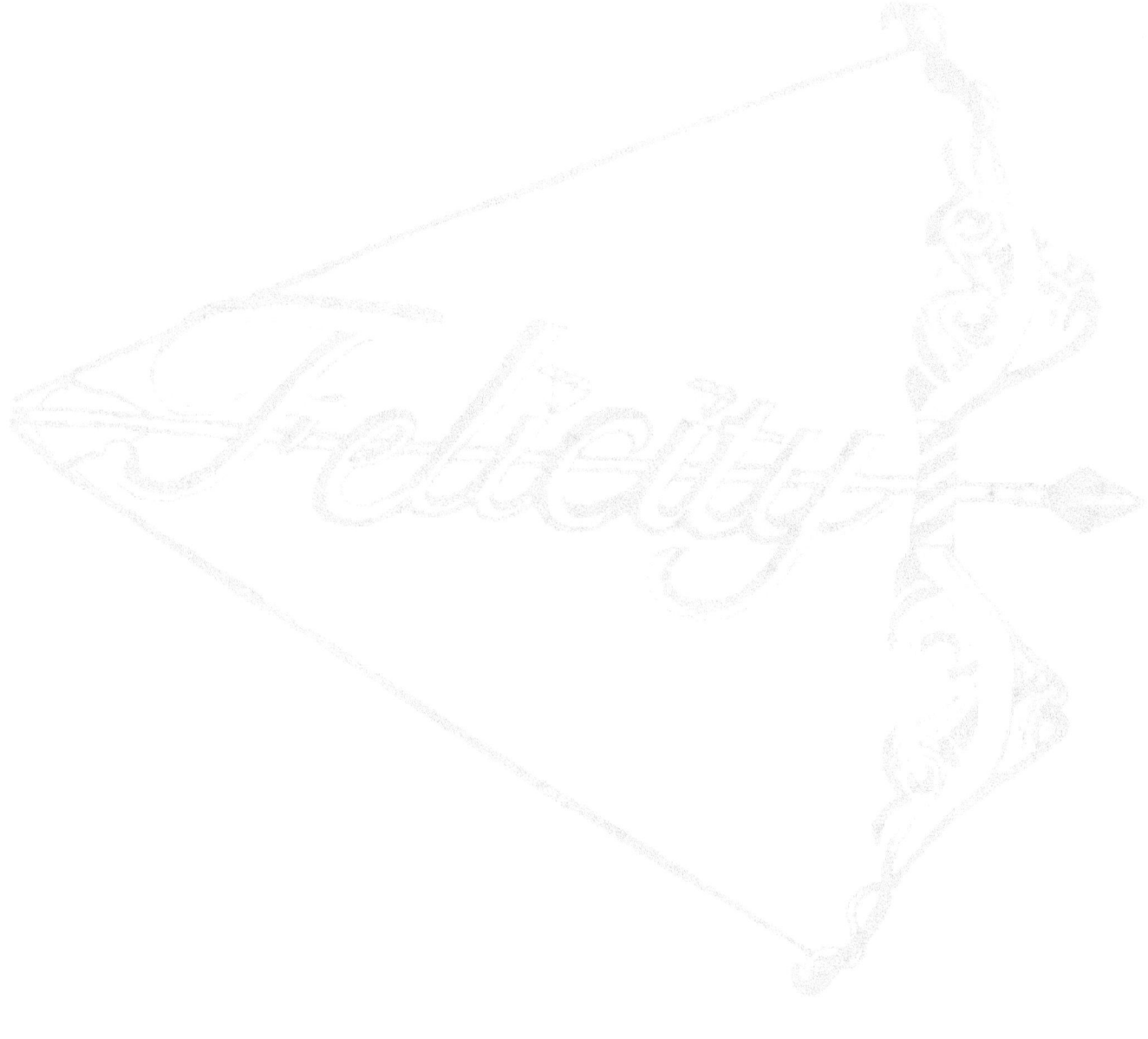

Apple Pork Tenderloin

Ingredients:

- 1 (2 lb) pork tenderloin
- 1 tsp garlic powder
- 1 medium white onion, chopped
- 1/3 cup honey
- 1 TBSP ground cinnamon
- Salt and pepper to taste
- 1 TBSP olive oil
- 2 large apples, peeled and chopped
- 2 cups chicken broth

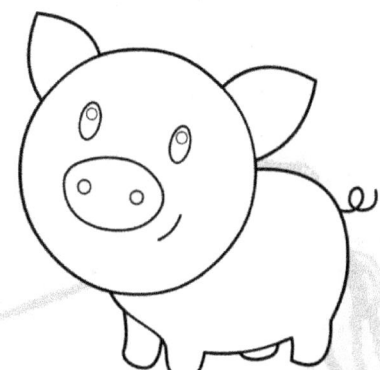

Directions:

1. Label gallon sized bag, "*Apple Pork Tenderloin*"
   +Add 2 cups chicken broth
   + Cook on low 8 hours"
2. In a medium mixing bowl, mix honey and olive oil together.
3. Stir garlic powder, cinnamon, salt, and pepper into honey mixture.
4. Add chopped onion and apples into your bowl.
5. Place tenderloin in your gallon sized bag first, then pour your apple-honey mixture over the meat.
6. Shake and roll sealed bag to mix ingredients.
7. Slightly open and squeeze bag to release as much excess air as possible, flattening meal for easier storage.
8. Freeze until you're ready to use.

Meal Idea: Serve over mashed cauliflower.

Rosemary Turkey Breast

Ingredients:

- 3-4 lb boneless turkey breast or 5-7 lb bone-in turkey breast
- 1 medium yellow onion, finely chopped
- 1 cup carrots, chopped
- 1 cup celery, chopped
- 2 TBSP garlic, finely minced
- 3 TBSP fresh rosemary, chopped
- 2 tsp poultry seasoning
- 1 tsp garlic powder
- 1 tsp onion powder
- 1 TBSP dried thyme
- 1 TBSP dried sage
- 2 cups chicken broth

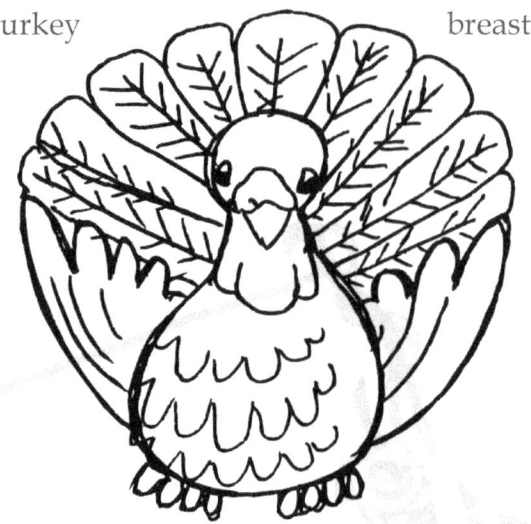

Directions:

1. For this freezer meal you will not unwrap your turkey breast until you are ready to use it. You will, however, prepare all other ingredients in 2 separate bags. Label 1 gallon sized bag and 1 quart sized bag.
   "Turkey Breast Veggies (gallon) and Turkey Breast herbs"
   + Place breast in crockpot with add chicken broth
   +Rub a portion of the herbs all over breast
   +Pour vegetables and remaining herbs in crockpot, around breast
   +Cook on low
     -Boneless=6-8 hours
     -Bone-in=8-10 hours
2. Place onion, celery, carrots, garlic, and 2 TBS rosemary in gallon sized bag.
3. Put remaining rosemary, poultry seasoning, garlic powder, onion powder, thyme, and sage in quart sized bag.
4. Shake and roll sealed bags to mix ingredients.
5. Slightly open and squeeze bags to release as much excess air as possible, flattening meal for easier storage.
6. Freeze until you're ready to use.

Place turkey breast in your refrigerator to thaw the day before you plan to prepare this meal.

BONUS: Serve your turkey breast with this delicious mashed cauliflower recipe.

Mashed Cauliflower

Ingredients:

- 1 head cauliflower
- 1 tsp garlic powder
- 1 TBS coconut oil
- ¼ cup unsweetened, original almond milk
- Salt and pepper to taste

Directions:

1. Rinse and chop cauliflower into florets.
2. Steam cauliflower florets for 10 minutes or until soft.
3. Put garlic powder, coconut oil, almond milk, salt, and pepper into food processor.
4. Pour hot, steamed cauliflower into food processor.
5. Pulse until cauliflower has a creamy texture.
6. Serve hot and enjoy!

If you do not have a food processor, you can use a mixer or mash cauliflower by hand

Eat Good–Feel Good
Dinner Recipes

'Who Needs Pasta?'-Spaghetti

Meat Sauce Ingredients:
- 2 lbs ground Italian sausage (or ground meat of your choice)
- 1 small yellow onion, finely chopped
- 2-3 cups tomato sauce
- 1 (14.5 oz) can diced tomatoes
- 1 TBS dried basil
- 1 TBS garlic, finely minced
- 2 tsp dried oregano
- 1 TBS Italian seasoning
- Salt and pepper to taste
- 1 TBS coconut

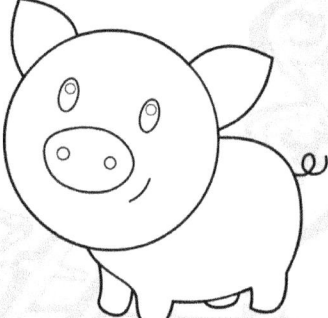

Garlic Spaghetti Squash Ingredients:
- 1 spaghetti squash
- 2 TBS coconut or olive oil
- 2 TBS garlic, finely minced
- 1 TBS fresh parsley, minced
- 1 small yellow onion, finely chopped
- Salt and pepper to taste

Directions:
1. Preheat oven to 400 degrees.
2. Place whole squash in preheated oven on a cookie sheet.
3. Set kitchen timer to bake squash for 45 minutes.
4. While squash in baking, prepare sauce.
5. In a large sauce pan combine tomato sauce, diced tomatoes, garlic, Italian seasoning, and salt. Cook over low-medium heat for 5 minutes.
6. In a large mixing bowl stir basil, oregano, salt, and pepper into ground pork or beef. You may have to use your hands.
7. Melt coconut oil in large skillet or frying pan and sauté onions on low heat for 1-2 minutes.
8. Add ground pork or beef to skillet and brown meat.

(Continued on Page 48)

9. When meat is completely cooked, strain excess fat and liquid.
10. Add meat to sauce pan. Cook on low for 10-15 minutes.
11. Take squash out of the oven and allow it to cool until you are able to hold it with your hands.
12. Cut squash in half lengthwise. Scoop all seeds out and discard.
13. Using a fork, scrape strand-like "pasta" from your squash. The squash should just come out. If it is difficult to scrape it out, return to the oven for an additional 10 minutes.
14. In a large skillet sauté onion, garlic, and parsley on medium heat for 2 minutes.
15. Add squash to skillet and sauté on low for 3 minutes, stirring occasionally.
16. Serve meat sauce over squash and enjoy!

Ham and Chicken Fried Rice

Ingredients:

- 1 head of cauliflower
- 2 (12.5 oz.) canned chicken in water
- 1 cup precooked ham, cut into small cubes
- 3 eggs
- ½ cup frozen peas
- ½ carrots, chopped
- 3 TBS green onion, finely chopped
- 3 TBS coconut aminos or soy sauce
- 2 TBS sesame oil
- 2 TBS olive oil
- 1 packet fried rice seasoning (I prefer the Sun-Bird brand)

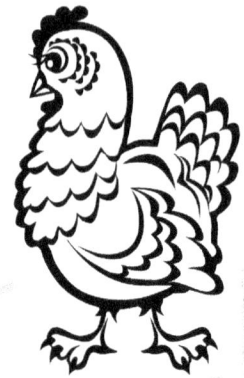

Directions:

1. Preheat oven to 375 degrees
2. Rinse and chop cauliflower into florets.
3. Place florets into a food processor and pulse until shredded, resembling rice. If you do not have a food processor, GET ONE! Until then, you can continue to chop your cauliflower manually until it resembles rice. Set aside.
4. In a large skillet sauté peas, carrots, and onion in sesame oil until they are tender. Pour vegetables and oil into a large mixing bowl.
5. Grease a smaller skillet with olive oil and cook the eggs, scrambling them with a spatula. Add the cooked eggs into the large mixing bowl.
6. Add the chicken, ham, and seasoning packet to the bowl, mixing all the ingredients together.
7. Mix the riced cauliflower and coconut aminos/soy sauce into the large mixing bowl.
8. Grease a metal cookie sheet with olive oil.
9. Spoon cauliflower rice mixture onto the cookie sheet, spreading it over the entire pan.
10. Bake for 15-20 minutes or until "rice" is at the texture you desire.
11. Cool and enjoy!

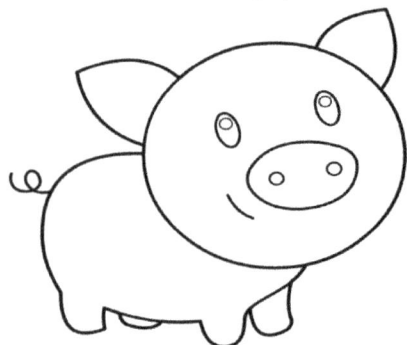

Bikini-Zucchini Boats

*Enjoy playing with different toppings for these fun,
unique recipe that your entire family will love!*

Pizza Boat

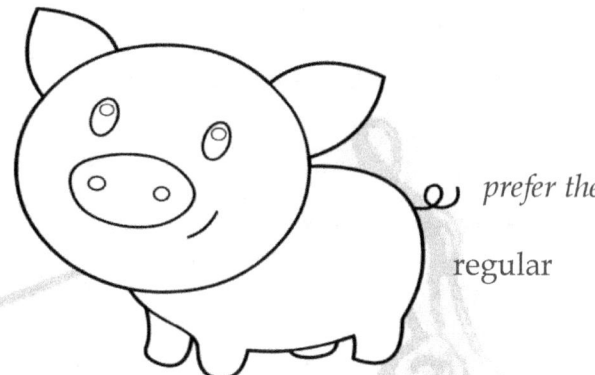

Ingredients:
- 3 medium-large zucchini
- 2 lbs ground Italian sausage
  -You can use plain ground sausage but I *prefer the*
  flavor and convenience of Italian sausage. regular
- 1 cup mini pepperoni slices or chopped
  pepperoni slices
- ½ cup marinara sauce
- 1 (14.5 oz.) can diced tomatoes, liquid drained
- 1 (2.25 oz.) can sliced black olives, liquid drained
- 1 small red onion, finely chopped
- ¼ cup bell pepper, chopped
- ¼ cup mushrooms, chopped
- 2 tsp Italian seasoning

Directions:
1. Preheat oven to 375 degrees.
2. Slice each zucchini in half lengthwise.
3. Using a metal spoon carefully scoop the inside of each zucchini out, leaving them "boat shaped" to fill in later.
4. Place halves on a cookie sheet and set aside for now.
5. In a large skillet brown sausage or pork. Drain excess liquid.
6. In a large mixing bowl stir together the marinara sauce, diced tomatoes, black olives, red onion, bell pepper, mushrooms, and Italian seasoning.
7. Add sausage and pepperoni slices to large mixing blown. Stir ingredients together.
8. Spoon meat mixture into the hollowed zucchini halves.
9. Place boats back on the cookie sheet and bake for 15-20 minutes.

Cool and enjoy!

Taco Boat

Ingredients:
- 3 medium-large zucchini
- 2 lbs ground beef
- 1 lime, juiced
- 1 small yellow onion, chopped
- 1 TBSP garlic, finely minced
- 1 TBSP olive oil
- ½ cup tomato sauce
- 1 (14.5 oz.) can diced tomatoes
- 1 (2.25 oz.) can diced green chilies
- Fresh cilantro to taste
- 1 taco seasoning packet
- 1 tsp dried oregano
- A pinch of cayenne pepper, to taste

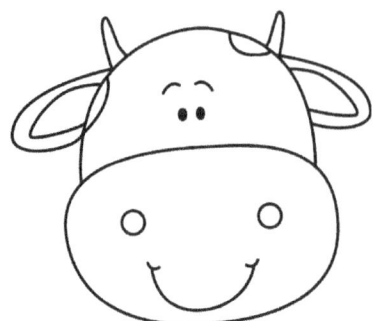

Directions:
1. Preheat oven to 375 degrees.
2. Slice each zucchini in half lengthwise.
3. Using a metal spoon carefully scoop the inside of each zucchini out, leaving them "boat shaped" to fill in later.
4. Place halves on a cookie sheet and set aside for now.
In a large skillet sauté onion, garlic, and fresh cilantro in olive oil for 2 minutes on medium heat.
5. Add ground beef to skillet and cook over medium heat until beef is thoroughly browned. Drain excess liquid.
6. In a large mixing bowl stir together the lime juice, tomato sauce, diced tomatoes, green chilies, taco seasoning, oregano, and cayenne pepper.
7. Add ground beef and sautéed vegetables to large mixing blown. Stir ingredients together.
8. Spoon meat mixture into the hollowed zucchini halves.
9. Place boats back on the cookie sheet and bake for 15-20 minutes.
10. Cool and enjoy!

Sweet and Spicy Glazed Salmon

Ingredients:
- 4 (4 oz.) skinless salmon fillets
- 2 limes
- 2 TBSP honey
- 2 TBSP olive oil
- 2 TBSP sugar free maple syrup
- 1 TBSP chili powder
- 2 tsp cumin
- Salt and pepper to taste
- ¼ tsp cayenne pepper (optional)

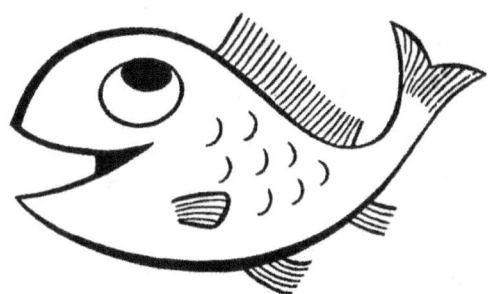

Directions:
1. Preheat oven to 400 degrees.
2. Line a shallow baking dish with tinfoil and grease it using olive or coconut oil.
3. Prepare glaze in a medium mixing bowl; stirring juice of 1 lime, honey, olive oil, syrup, chili powder, cumin, salt, pepper, and cayenne pepper together.
4. Place salmon fillets in greased baking dish.
5. Brush and/or rub glaze over salmon.
6. Cut remaining lime into quarter wedges. Squeeze some juice from them over salmon and place them inside the baking dish.
7. Bake for 10 minutes. Carefully turn fillets over and brush glaze mixture onto the other side of them.
8. Bake an additional 15 minutes.
9. Cool and ENJOY!

No-Bun Burgers

Ingredients:

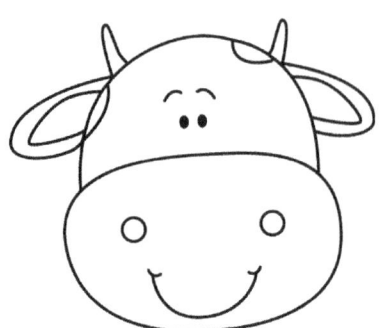

- 3 lbs ground beef
- 1 TBSP garlic, finely minced
- 2 TBSP white onion, finely minced
- 1 (1 oz.) ranch seasoning packet
- 2 tsp garlic powder
- 2 TBSP onion soup mix
- 2 tsp black pepper
- 2 tsp paprika
- 1 TBSP season salt

Directions:

1. Lay a sheet of parchment paper on clean counter surface to place patties on later.
2. In large mixing bowl combine all dry seasonings; ranch packet, garlic powder, onion soup mix, paprika, pepper, and season salt.
3. Add beef, garlic, and onion to the mixing bowl. Using your hands, mix everything into the meat.
4. Form patties with your hands, flattening them to your desired thickness.
5. Season with desired amount of salt and pepper on both sides of each patty.
6. Place each patty on prepared parchment sheet.
7. To freeze; cut parchment paper in squares around each patty and stake them on top of each other with 1 sheet of paper between patties. Label gallon sized bag and place stacked patties inside. Squeeze as much air out of the bag as you can and freeze.
8. To cook; Grill, broil, or fry patties on stovetop until they're cooked thoroughly.
9. Lay large pieces of iceberg or romaine lettuce on a plate, you will use this to wrap around your burger (and you won't even miss the bun).
10. Get creative and add delicious Paleo toppings to your lettuce wrap.
11. Place cooked burger on top of the toppings you've selected, tightly wrap the lettuce around your burger, and ENJOY this guilt free burger!

Voyage: Workbook
London Solomon

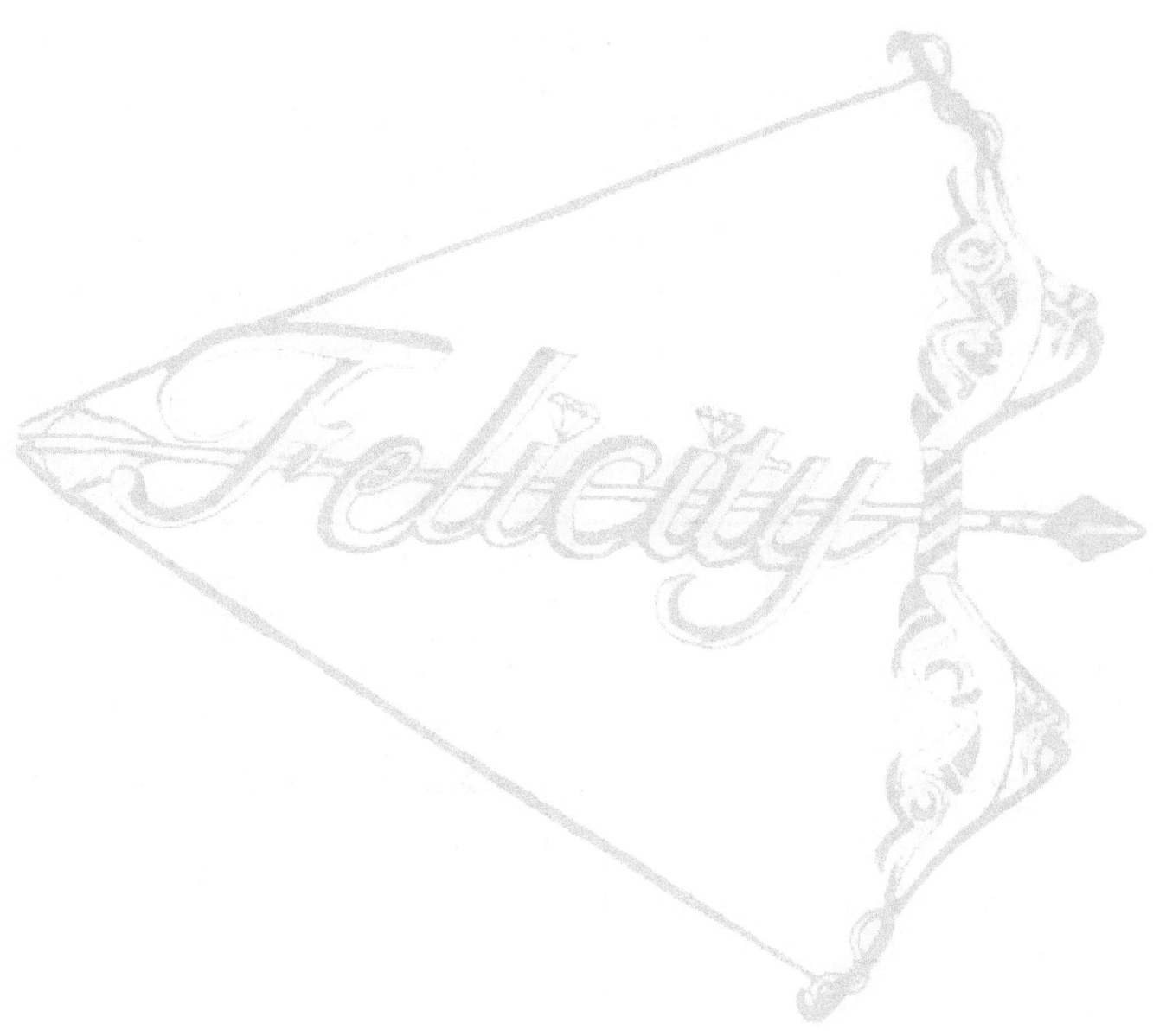

Let's Put Your Meal Plan Together

I have compiled a small list of side and snack ideas. You are not, by any means, restricted to these foods. I just wanted to give you a few ideas that you could choose from when putting your meal plan together.

Vegetables

• Cauliflower	• Asparagus	• Cucumber
• Carrots	• Broccoli	• Zucchini
• Celery	• Green Beans	• Squash
• Tomatoes	• Peppers	• Sweet Potatoes
• Spinach	• Brussels Sprouts	• Eggplant
• Lettuce/Salad	• Cabbage	• Pumpkin
• Mushrooms		

Fruits

• Apples	• Strawberries
• Bananas	• Raspberries
• Grapefruit	• Blueberries
• Oranges	• Melons
• Pineapple	• Lemons
• Peaches	• Limes

Healthy Fats

Avocados	Olives	Nuts and Seeds	Nut Butters	Oils

Ready or Not, It's Time to Change Your Life!

Remember this example that you saw earlier? Take a second look and think about what you would like your own to look like. If you're still not sure exactly how to plan your day, don't be afraid to look back to subjects that you may have a difficult time remembering.

	Monday
Water	[ ] 20 oz. [ ] 20 oz. [ ] 20 oz. [ ] 20 oz. [ ] 20 oz. [ ] 20 oz. = 120 oz.
Breakfast	*2 fried eggs, 2 strips of bacon, 1 cup strawberries*
Snack	*Cucumber slices*
Lunch	*Turkey wrap with cashews*
Snack	*Apple*
Dinner	*Avocado double burger with sweet potato fries*
Exercise?	*Walked 1 mile at 7 pm*

Be sure to read the description of the worksheets I've provided for your next 30 days BEFORE you begin. It is vital that you understand how and why it is so important for you to consistently follow these worksheets if you plan to be successful!

I have done my best to provide you with all the tools you will need for the first 30 days of your new life. Use them, take advantage of all that this book has to offer, and set yourself up for success in the very beginning by making a commitment to yourself and follow through with this plan for 30 days. You can do anything for 30 days … but I promise you that if you stick with it, you'll never go back to living any other way.

Worksheet Breakdown

Worksheet #1:

Goals for My First 30 Days of Paleo

Let's start working through your worksheets so that you have a better understanding of how they can help you. The first worksheet you will find is the Goals for My First 30 Days of Paleo. This is the only worksheet with only one copy in the book and it only has space for three goals. The simplicity of this worksheet was intentional. After each of the three goals, you are asked to answer the question:

"What steps am I going to take to achieve this goal?"

Before starting to fill out your worksheets, think long and hard about this one. It is the first worksheet because it is the most important.

Specify exactly what you will work to accomplish physically in 30 days. Set appropriate expectations. You will not lose 100 pounds in 30 days. If that is your goal, you will fail. Set goals you feel confident that you can achieve with extra work.

When setting your last two goals spend a little time soul searching and really find a meaningful goal that will force you to work on yourself as a person, rather than a body. If you are open to it, this lifestyle can offer you an opportunity for profound spiritual growth and an opportunity to get to explore yourself on a much deeper psychological level.

Once you have come up with your three goals put a lot of thought into the steps you will have to take to achieve your goals. Write what you need to do, what you need to change, and why you know you will succeed. Throughout your first 30 days, refer back to this page frequently to remind yourself what you're working for.

Worksheet #2:

Weekly Success Plan

This worksheet is intended to be filled out prior to the upcoming week (I like to do my meal prep and planning Sundays but any day is fine as everyone's schedules are different). Plan on spending about an hour just filling this worksheet out and planning your meals and activity for the week.

You will use this worksheet to log your meals, exercise, and water intake for each day of the week. Keeping an honest and detailed record of what you eat will help you tremendously throughout this journey. Don't cheat yourself by skipping these logs or not recording everything you eat. No one is perfect and there may be times that you slip up and eat something that isn't necessarily good for you. Write it down and move on. Do not dwell on little slip ups, feel guilty, get upset with yourself, or pretend they didn't happen by not writing them in your log. There's no shame in being imperfect but by tracking every single thing you eat, you are holding yourself accountable and will feel motivated to stay on track. These worksheets are designed for YOU and only you. I have included them in this book to make this lifestyle change easier for beginners. Take advantage of the tools available here. If you choose not to, you are the only person it will affect.

Worksheet #3:

Meal Plan Grocery List

If I haven't pounded the importance of preparedness and planning enough yet, let me express how strongly I feel about preparation:

IF YOU DO NOT WANT TO FAIL - EVERY SINGLE WEEK YOU <u>MUST</u> WRITE A MEAL PLAN, WRITE A DETAILED GROCERY LIST TO INCLUDE ALL THE ITEMS ON YOUR MEAL PLAN AND SHOP. SPEND AT LEAST AN HOUR IN THE KITCHEN EVERY WEEK PREPARING YOUR FOOD.

- Follow your meal plan
- Drink your water
- Fuel your mind, body and soul with beautiful, natural foods
- Think positive thoughts and spend some time getting to know you

Not only are you capable of achieving your goals, you DESERVE it!

Now that we've got that out of the way, let's talk about the grocery list for your weekly meal plan. It is SO important that you plan your entire week's meals and put that time in the kitchen doing food prep, especially when you're a beginner. If your food is ready and available when you're hungry, you're much more likely to stick to your meal plan. I understand that it all seems like so much work, and at first it will be, but when you're enjoying the endless benefits of a body fueled by REAL, natural, nutritious food-you will begin to enjoy the process.

Worksheet #4:

Daily Log and Journal Entry

On the next 2 pages you will find a daily log worksheet and journal space. This worksheet is broken down into 5 sections:

1. The A.M. section is for you to write the date, day number (which day you are on in your journey), and how many hours of sleep you got the night before. Just below the A.M .section there is a place that you can write your morning weight-your starting weight=thee amount of weight you have lost total. *THIS PORTION OF THE WORKSHEET IS ABSOLUTELY OPTIONAL!* Some people find daily weights motivating, but I typically suggest you only weigh yourself weekly.

2. There are 6 boxed with "20 oz." inside of them. These are intended to be crossed off as you drink your water throughout the day. I cannot stress enough how important it is that you drink all 120 ounces of water every single day.

3. Next is your daily food log. This is where you will write down what you've eaten for the day. I find that logs are more accurate if they are filled out throughout the day, as you eat, rather than at the end of the day because we have a tendency to forget the little things.

4. I feel most strongly about 100% completion of the P.M. section for at least 30 days but would suggest practicing this habit every day for the rest of your life.

This is where you are to write at least three things you love about yourself. Don't get so wrapped up in what you're trying to change about yourself that you forget what an incredible human you already are.

5. Lastly, I have included a little over a page of space for you to journal every day. You can write about anything but it is beneficial to include a little note about how you're feeling physically and emotionally about the way you're eating. Journaling is incredibly therapeutic and this lifestyle change isn't just about losing weight or making ourselves look a different way. I hope you use this opportunity to grow spiritually as well.

Keeping an honest and detailed record of what you eat will help you tremendously throughout this journey. Don't cheat yourself by skipping these logs or not recording everything you eat. No one is perfect and there may be times that you slip up and eat something that isn't necessarily good for you. Write it down and move on. Do not dwell on little slip ups, feel guilty, get upset with yourself, or pretend they didn't happen by not writing them in your log. There's no shame in "falling off the wagon" but by tracking every single thing you eat, you are holding yourself accountable and will feel motivated to stay on track. These worksheets are designed for YOU and only you. I have included them in this book to make this lifestyle change easier for beginners. Take advantage of the tools available here. If you choose not to, you are only cheating yourself.

I've given you a lot of information. Expect to spend a little time re-reading a few things. It has been over 2 years since I embarked on this journey and I am still constantly learning. Keep in mind that when you purchased this book and made the incredible decision to embark on this "voyage", you also became a part of the Felicity family. Below you will find 30 days' worth of worksheets to make the beginning
of your journey as simple as possible. Use the tools inside this book because they were created to ensure your success.

We are here to help, guide, and support you any way that we can. If you are on Facebook, be sure to like our page for fun new recipes, tips and tricks, DIY beauty and self-care regimens, health and wellness product reviews (including discount codes), support and encouragement from incredible people on the same journey as you are, and lots of laughs. You are also welcome to message me directly with any questions, concerns, or struggles you might be having. This isn't just another "cookbook" or "diet manual." I've poured my heart and soul into this book and my company, Felicity, because it is my passion to share the invaluable information about the Paleo lifestyle with others because it truly changed, possibly even saved my life.

www.facebook.com/felicitylondonsolomon

There are simply no words to express my gratitude for your faith in me and your interest in my work and the Paleo lifestyle. I truly put my heart and soul into this book because I am so passionate about sharing this incredible life-changing journey I've taken on.

I am truly so very excited for you to begin and very sincerely care about your own personal path. As I wrote above, I am not only the author, but I would like to be your friend, support system, and cheerleader if you'll let me by sharing your story. I know you will see miraculous changes in your body and mind soon. You will be successful because you deserve this! The best of luck to you!

Keep an eye out for other books and products brought to you by Felicity.
We have only just begun.
Voyage Workbook

Goals for My First 30 Days Paleo

Goal #1: _____
The steps I am going to take to achieve this goal:

_____

_____

_____

_____

Goal #2: _____
The steps I am going to take to achieve this goal:

_____

_____

_____

_____

Goal #3: _____
The steps I am going to take to achieve this goal:

_____

_____

_____

_____

Weekly Success Plan
Week

	Breakfast	Snack	Lunch	Snack	Dinner	Exercise
M Day #__ Date:						
T Day #__ Date:						
W Day #__ Date:						
T Day #__ Date:						
F Day #__ Date:						
S Day #__ Date:						
S Day #__ Date:						

Meal Plan Grocery List

Week _/_/__ - _/_/__

Monday	Tuesday	Wednesday	Thursday	Friday	Saturday	Sunday	Healthy Snacks

 **AM Log**

Date: Day: Hours of Sleep:

Morning Weight: ▭   Start Weight: ▤   Weight Lost

H2O CHECK-OFF

| 20 Ounces | 20 Ounces | 20 Ounces |
| 20 Ounces | 20 Ounces | 20 Ounces |

FO OD

LOG

Breakfast	Snack	Lunch	Snack	Dinner

 **PM Log**

3 Things I Love About Me Today

 #1: _____

 #2: _____

 #3: _____

Daily Journal Entry:

AM Log

Date: Day: Hours of Sleep:

Morning Weight: Start Weight: Weight Lost

H2O CHECK-OFF

| 20 Ounces | 20 Ounces | 20 Ounces |
| 20 Ounces | 20 Ounces | 20 Ounces |

FO OD

LOG

Breakfast	Snack	Lunch	Snack	Dinner

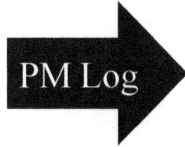

PM Log

3 Things I Love About Me Today

 #1: _____

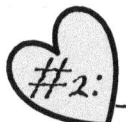 #2: _____

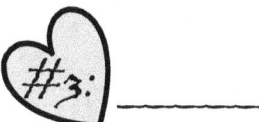 #3: _____

Daily Journal Entry:

AM Log

Date: Day: Hours of Sleep:

Morning Weight: ⬭ Start Weight: ⬒ Weight Lost

H20 **CHECK-OFF**

| 20 Ounces | 20 Ounces | 20 Ounces |
| 20 Ounces | 20 Ounces | 20 Ounces |

FO OD

LOG

Breakfast	Snack	Lunch	Snack	Dinner

PM Log

3 Things I Love About Me Today

 #1: _____

 #2: _____

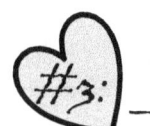 #3: _____

Daily Journal Entry:

_____

_____

_____

_____

_____

_____

_____

_____

_____

_____

_____

_____

_____

_____

_____

_____

 **AM Log**

Date: Day: Hours of Sleep:

Morning Weight: Start Weight: Weight Lost

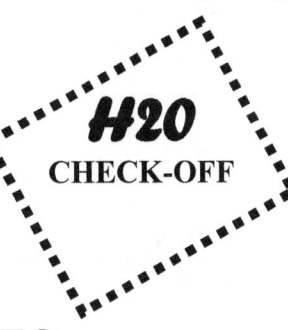

H20 CHECK-OFF

| 20 Ounces | 20 Ounces | 20 Ounces |
| 20 Ounces | 20 Ounces | 20 Ounces |

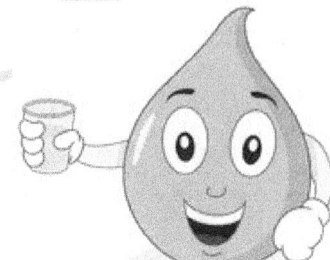

FO OD

LOG

Breakfast	Snack	Lunch	Snack	Dinner

 **PM Log**

3 Things I Love About Me Today

 #1: _____

 #2: _____

 #3: _____

Daily Journal Entry:

_____

_____

_____

_____

_____

_____

_____

_____

_____

_____

_____

_____

_____

_____

_____

_____

_____

_____

AM Log

Date: Day: Hours of Sleep:

Morning Weight: ⬭ Start Weight: ⊟ Weight Lost

H20 CHECK-OFF

| 20 Ounces | 20 Ounces | 20 Ounces |
| 20 Ounces | 20 Ounces | 20 Ounces |

FO OD

LOG

Breakfast	Snack	Lunch	Snack	Dinner

PM Log

3 Things I Love About Me Today

 #1: _____    #2: _____    #3: _____

Daily Journal Entry:

 **AM Log**

Date: Day: Hours of Sleep:

Morning Weight: ▭ Start Weight: ▤ Weight Lost

H20 **CHECK-OFF**

20 Ounces	20 Ounces	20 Ounces
20 Ounces	20 Ounces	20 Ounces

FOOD

LOG

Breakfast	Snack	Lunch	Snack	Dinner

 **PM Log**

3 Things I Love About Me Today

 #1: _____

 #2: _____

 #3: _____

Daily Journal Entry:

_____

_____

_____

_____

_____

_____

_____

_____

_____

_____

_____

_____

_____

_____

_____

_____

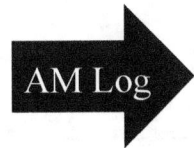 **AM Log**

Date: Day: Hours of Sleep:

Morning Weight: ▭ Start Weight: ▤ Weight Lost

H2O CHECK-OFF

20 Ounces	20 Ounces	20 Ounces
20 Ounces	20 Ounces	20 Ounces

FOOD

LOG

Breakfast	Snack	Lunch	Snack	Dinner

 **PM Log**

3 Things I Love About Me Today

 #1: _____    #2: _____   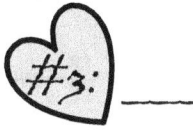 #3: _____

Daily Journal Entry:

_____

_____

_____

_____

_____

_____

_____

_____

_____

_____

_____

_____

_____

_____

_____

_____

Meal Plan Grocery List

Week _ / / _ - _ / / _

Monday	Tuesday	Wednesday	Thursday	Friday	Saturday	Sunday	Healthy Snacks

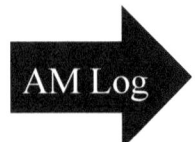
AM Log

Date: Day: Hours of Sleep:

Morning Weight: ▭ Start Weight: ▤ Weight Lost

H2O CHECK-OFF

| 20 Ounces | 20 Ounces | 20 Ounces |
| 20 Ounces | 20 Ounces | 20 Ounces |

FO OD

LOG

Breakfast	Snack	Lunch	Snack	Dinner

PM Log

3 Things I Love About Me Today

 #1: _____

 #2: _____

 #3: _____

Daily Journal Entry:

_____

_____

_____

_____

_____

_____

_____

_____

_____

_____

_____

_____

_____

_____

_____

_____

 **AM Log**

Date: Day: Hours of Sleep:

Morning Weight: ▬ Start Weight: ▤ Weight Lost

H2O CHECK-OFF

| 20 Ounces | 20 Ounces | 20 Ounces |
| 20 Ounces | 20 Ounces | 20 Ounces |

FO OD

LOG

Breakfast	Snack	Lunch	Snack	Dinner

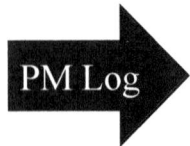 **PM Log**

3 Things I Love About Me Today

 #1: _____    #2: _____    #3: _____

Daily Journal Entry:

_____

_____

_____

_____

_____

_____

_____

_____

_____

_____

_____

_____

_____

_____

_____

AM Log

Date: Day: Hours of Sleep:

Morning Weight: ⬛ Start Weight: ⬛ Weight Lost

H2O CHECK-OFF

| 20 Ounces | 20 Ounces | 20 Ounces |
| 20 Ounces | 20 Ounces | 20 Ounces |

FO
OD

LOG

Breakfast	Snack	Lunch	Snack	Dinner

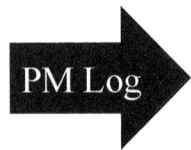

PM Log

3 Things I Love About Me Today

 #1: _____

 #2: _____

 #3: _____

Daily Journal Entry:

_____

_____

_____

_____

_____

_____

_____

_____

_____

_____

_____

_____

_____

_____

_____

_____

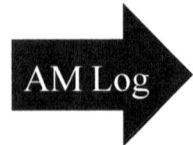

AM Log

Date: Day: Hours of Sleep:

Morning Weight: ▭ Start Weight: ▤ Weight Lost

H2O CHECK-OFF

20 Ounces	20 Ounces	20 Ounces
20 Ounces	20 Ounces	20 Ounces

FO OD

LOG

Breakfast	Snack	Lunch	Snack	Dinner

PM Log

3 Things I Love About Me Today

 #1: _____

 #2: _____

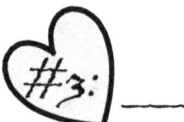 #3: _____

Daily Journal Entry:

 **AM Log**

Date: Day: Hours of Sleep:

Morning Weight: ⬜ Start Weight: ⬛ Weight Lost

H2O CHECK-OFF

20 Ounces	20 Ounces	20 Ounces
20 Ounces	20 Ounces	20 Ounces

FOOD

LOG

Breakfast	Snack	Lunch	Snack	Dinner

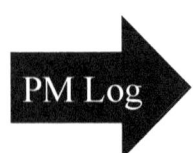 **PM Log**

3 Things I Love About Me Today

 #1: _____    #2: _____   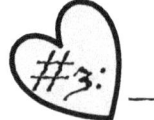 #3: _____

Daily Journal Entry:

_____

_____

_____

_____

_____

_____

_____

_____

_____

_____

_____

_____

_____

_____

_____

AM Log

Date: Day: Hours of Sleep:

Morning Weight: ⊟ Start Weight: ☰ Weight Lost

H2O **CHECK-OFF**

| 20 Ounces | 20 Ounces | 20 Ounces |
| 20 Ounces | 20 Ounces | 20 Ounces |

FO
OD

LOG

Breakfast	Snack	Lunch	Snack	Dinner

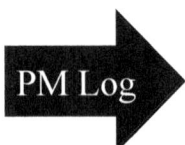
PM Log

3 Things I Love About Me Today

#1: _____

#2: _____

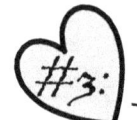
#3: _____

Daily Journal Entry:

AM Log

Date: Day: Hours of Sleep:

Morning Weight: ▭   Start Weight: ⊟   Weight Lost

H2O CHECK-OFF

| 20 Ounces | 20 Ounces | 20 Ounces |
| 20 Ounces | 20 Ounces | 20 Ounces |

FO OD

LOG

Breakfast	Snack	Lunch	Snack	Dinner

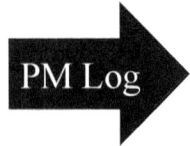

PM Log

3 Things I Love About Me Today

 #1: _____

 #2: _____

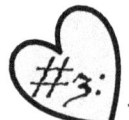 #3: _____

Daily Journal Entry:

_____

_____

_____

_____

_____

_____

_____

_____

_____

_____

_____

_____

_____

_____

_____

_____

_____

Meal Plan Grocery List

Week _ / _ / _ _ - _ / _ / _ _

Monday	Tuesday	Wednesday	Thursday	Friday	Saturday	Sunday	Healthy Snacks

AM Log

Date: Day: Hours of Sleep:

Morning Weight: Start Weight: Weight Lost

H2O CHECK-OFF

20 Ounces	20 Ounces	20 Ounces
20 Ounces	20 Ounces	20 Ounces

FOOD

LOG

Breakfast	Snack	Lunch	Snack	Dinner

PM Log

3 Things I Love About Me Today

 #1: _____

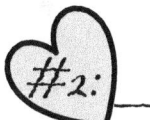 #2: _____

 #3: _____

Daily Journal Entry:

 **AM Log**

Date: Day: Hours of Sleep:

Morning Weight: ▭ Start Weight: ⬒ Weight Lost

H2O CHECK-OFF

| 20 Ounces | 20 Ounces | 20 Ounces |
| 20 Ounces | 20 Ounces | 20 Ounces |

FO OD

LOG

Breakfast	Snack	Lunch	Snack	Dinner

 **PM Log**

3 Things I Love About Me Today

 #1: _____

 #2: _____

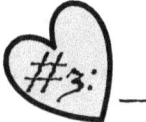 #3: _____

Daily Journal Entry:

_____

_____

_____

_____

_____

_____

_____

_____

_____

_____

_____

_____

_____

_____

 **AM Log**

Date: _____   Day: _____   Hours of Sleep: _____

Morning Weight: _____ ▭ Start Weight: _____ ▤ Weight Lost

H2O CHECK-OFF

| 20 Ounces | 20 Ounces | 20 Ounces |
| 20 Ounces | 20 Ounces | 20 Ounces |

FO
OD

LOG

Breakfast	Snack	Lunch	Snack	Dinner

 **PM Log**

3 Things I Love About Me Today

 #1: _____

 #2: _____

 #3: _____

Daily Journal Entry:

_____

_____

_____

_____

_____

_____

_____

_____

_____

_____

_____

_____

_____

_____

_____

AM Log

Date: Day: Hours of Sleep:

Morning Weight: ▭ Start Weight: ▤ Weight Lost

H2O
CHECK-OFF

| 20 Ounces | 20 Ounces | 20 Ounces |
| 20 Ounces | 20 Ounces | 20 Ounces |

FO
OD

LOG

Breakfast	Snack	Lunch	Snack	Dinner

PM Log

3 Things I Love About Me Today

 #1: _____

 #2: _____

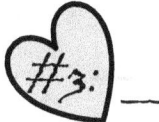 #3: _____

Daily Journal Entry:

_____

_____

_____

_____

_____

_____

_____

_____

_____

_____

_____

_____

_____

_____

_____

AM Log

Date: Day: Hours of Sleep:

Morning Weight: ▬ Start Weight: ▤ Weight Lost

H2O CHECK-OFF

| 20 Ounces | 20 Ounces | 20 Ounces |
| 20 Ounces | 20 Ounces | 20 Ounces |

FO OD

LOG

Breakfast	Snack	Lunch	Snack	Dinner

PM Log

3 Things I Love About Me Today

 #1: _____

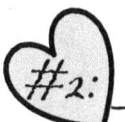 #2: _____

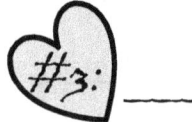 #3: _____

Daily Journal Entry:

AM Log

Date: Day: Hours of Sleep:

Morning Weight: ⬭ Start Weight: ▤ Weight Lost

H2O CHECK-OFF

| 20 Ounces | 20 Ounces | 20 Ounces |
| 20 Ounces | 20 Ounces | 20 Ounces |

FO
OD

LOG

Breakfast	Snack	Lunch	Snack	Dinner

PM Log

3 Things I Love About Me Today

 #1: _____

 #2: _____

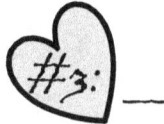 #3: _____

Daily Journal Entry:

_____

_____

_____

_____

_____

_____

_____

_____

_____

_____

_____

_____

_____

_____

_____

AM Log

Date: Day: Hours of Sleep:

Morning Weight: ▭ Start Weight: ▤ Weight Lost

H20 CHECK-OFF

| 20 Ounces | 20 Ounces | 20 Ounces |
| 20 Ounces | 20 Ounces | 20 Ounces |

FO
OD

LOG

Breakfast	Snack	Lunch	Snack	Dinner

PM Log

3 Things I Love About Me Today

 #1: _____

 #2: _____

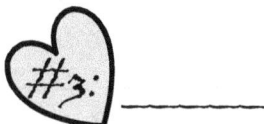 #3: _____

Daily Journal Entry:

_____

_____

_____

_____

_____

_____

_____

_____

_____

_____

_____

_____

_____

_____

Meal Plan Grocery List

Week _ / /__ - _ / /__

Monday	Tuesday	Wednesday	Thursday	Friday	Saturday	Sunday	Healthy Snacks

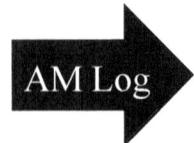 **AM Log**

Date: Day: Hours of Sleep:

Morning Weight: Start Weight: Weight Lost

H2O CHECK-OFF

| 20 Ounces | 20 Ounces | 20 Ounces |
| 20 Ounces | 20 Ounces | 20 Ounces |

FO OD

LOG

Breakfast	Snack	Lunch	Snack	Dinner

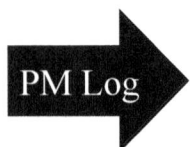 **PM Log**

3 Things I Love About Me Today

 #1: _____

 #2: _____

 #3: _____

Daily Journal Entry:

_____

_____

_____

_____

_____

_____

_____

_____

_____

_____

_____

_____

_____

_____

_____

AM Log

Date: Day: Hours of Sleep:

Morning Weight: ▭ Start Weight: ⊟ Weight Lost

H20 **CHECK-OFF**

| 20 Ounces | 20 Ounces | 20 Ounces |
| 20 Ounces | 20 Ounces | 20 Ounces |

FO OD

LOG

Breakfast	Snack	Lunch	Snack	Dinner

PM Log

3 Things I Love About Me Today

 #1: _____

 #2: _____

 #3: _____

Daily Journal Entry:

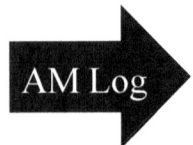 **AM Log**

Date: _____   Day: _____   Hours of Sleep: _____

Morning Weight: _____ ▭ Start Weight: _____ ▤ Weight Lost

H2O CHECK-OFF

| 20 Ounces | 20 Ounces | 20 Ounces |
| 20 Ounces | 20 Ounces | 20 Ounces |

FO OD

LOG

Breakfast	Snack	Lunch	Snack	Dinner

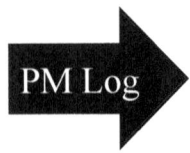 **PM Log**

3 Things I Love About Me Today

 #1: _____    #2: _____    #3: _____

Daily Journal Entry:

_____

_____

_____

_____

_____

_____

_____

_____

_____

_____

_____

_____

_____

_____

_____

_____

_____

AM Log

Date: Day: Hours of Sleep:

Morning Weight: ▭ Start Weight: ▤ Weight Lost

H2O
CHECK-OFF

| 20 Ounces | 20 Ounces | 20 Ounces |
| 20 Ounces | 20 Ounces | 20 Ounces |

FO
OD

LOG

Breakfast	Snack	Lunch	Snack	Dinner

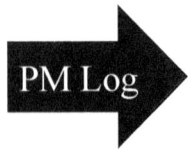

PM Log

3 Things I Love About Me Today

 #1: _____    #2: _____    #3: _____

Daily Journal Entry:

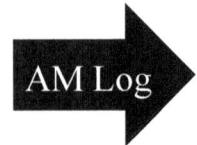 **AM Log**

Date: Day: Hours of Sleep:

Morning Weight: ▭ Start Weight: ⬒ Weight Lost

H2O CHECK-OFF

| 20 Ounces | 20 Ounces | 20 Ounces |

| 20 Ounces | 20 Ounces | 20 Ounces |

FOOD

LOG

Breakfast	Snack	Lunch	Snack	Dinner

 **PM Log**

3 Things I Love About Me Today

 #1: _____

 #2: _____

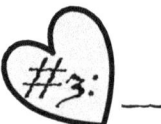 #3: _____

Daily Journal Entry:

_____

_____

_____

_____

_____

_____

_____

_____

_____

_____

_____

_____

_____

_____

_____

_____

Date: Day: Hours of Sleep:

Morning Weight: ▭ Start Weight: ▤ Weight Lost

H20 CHECK-OFF

| 20 Ounces | 20 Ounces | 20 Ounces |
| 20 Ounces | 20 Ounces | 20 Ounces |

FO
OD

LOG

Breakfast	Snack	Lunch	Snack	Dinner

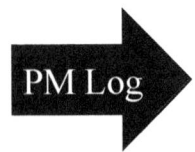

3 Things I Love About Me Today

 #1: _____

 #2: _____

 #3: _____

Daily Journal Entry:

_____

_____

_____

_____

_____

_____

_____

_____

_____

_____

_____

_____

_____

_____

_____

_____

AM Log

Date: Day: Hours of Sleep:

Morning Weight: ▭ Start Weight: ▤ Weight Lost

H20 CHECK-OFF

20 Ounces	20 Ounces	20 Ounces
20 Ounces	20 Ounces	20 Ounces

FO OD

LOG

Breakfast	Snack	Lunch	Snack	Dinner

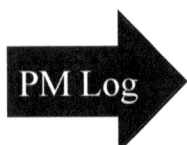

PM Log

3 Things I Love About Me Today

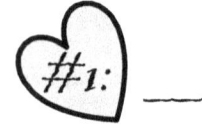 #1: _____

 #2: _____

 #3: _____

Daily Journal Entry:

Meal Plan Grocery List

Week __/__/__ - __/__/__

Monday	Tuesday	Wednesday	Thursday	Friday	Saturday	Sunday	Healthy Snacks

 AM Log

Date: Day: Hours of Sleep:

Morning Weight: ▭ Start Weight: ▤ Weight Lost

H2O CHECK-OFF

| 20 Ounces | 20 Ounces | 20 Ounces |
| 20 Ounces | 20 Ounces | 20 Ounces |

FO
OD

LOG

Breakfast	Snack	Lunch	Snack	Dinner

 PM Log

3 Things I Love About Me Today

 #1: _____

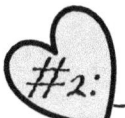 #2: _____

 #3: _____

Daily Journal Entry:

_____

_____

_____

_____

_____

_____

_____

_____

_____

_____

_____

_____

_____

_____

_____

_____

_____

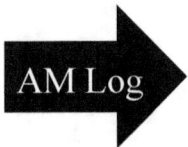

AM Log

Date: _____   Day: _____   Hours of Sleep: _____

Morning Weight: _____   ▭ Start Weight: _____   ▭ Weight Lost

H2O CHECK-OFF

| 20 Ounces | 20 Ounces | 20 Ounces |
| 20 Ounces | 20 Ounces | 20 Ounces |

FO
OD

LOG

Breakfast	Snack	Lunch	Snack	Dinner

PM Log

3 Things I Love About Me Today

 #1: _____

 #2: _____

 #3: _____

Daily Journal Entry:

_____

_____

_____

_____

_____

_____

_____

_____

_____

_____

_____

_____

_____

_____

_____

_____

_____

AM Log

Date: Day: Hours of Sleep:

Morning Weight: Start Weight: Weight Lost

H20 CHECK-OFF

| 20 Ounces | 20 Ounces | 20 Ounces |
| 20 Ounces | 20 Ounces | 20 Ounces |

FOOD

LOG

Breakfast	Snack	Lunch	Snack	Dinner

PM Log

3 Things I Love About Me Today

 #1: _____

 #2: _____

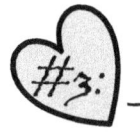 #3: _____

Daily Journal Entry:

_____

_____

_____

_____

_____

_____

_____

_____

_____

_____

_____

_____

_____

_____

_____

_____

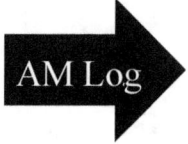

AM Log

Date: Day: Hours of Sleep:

Morning Weight: ▭ Start Weight: ▤ Weight Lost

H20 CHECK-OFF

| 20 Ounces | 20 Ounces | 20 Ounces |
| 20 Ounces | 20 Ounces | 20 Ounces |

FO OD

LOG

Breakfast	Snack	Lunch	Snack	Dinner

PM Log

3 Things I Love About Me Today

 #1: _____

 #2: _____

 #3: _____

Daily Journal Entry:

_____

_____

_____

_____

_____

_____

_____

_____

_____

_____

_____

_____

_____

_____

_____

_____

 **AM Log**

Date: Day: Hours of Sleep:

Morning Weight: ⬜   Start Weight: ⬜   Weight Lost

H2O CHECK-OFF

| 20 Ounces | 20 Ounces | 20 Ounces |
| 20 Ounces | 20 Ounces | 20 Ounces |

FOOD

LOG

Breakfast	Snack	Lunch	Snack	Dinner

PM Log

3 Things I Love About Me Today

 #1: _____

 #2: _____

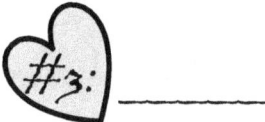 #3: _____

Daily Journal Entry:

_____

_____

_____

_____

_____

_____

_____

_____

_____

_____

_____

_____

_____

_____

_____

 **AM Log**

Date: Day: Hours of Sleep:

Morning Weight: ⬛ Start Weight: ☰ Weight Lost

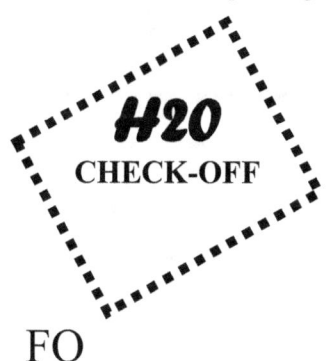

| 20 Ounces | 20 Ounces | 20 Ounces |
| 20 Ounces | 20 Ounces | 20 Ounces |

H2O CHECK-OFF

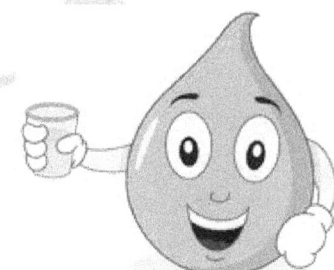

FO OD

LOG

Breakfast	Snack	Lunch	Snack	Dinner

 **PM Log**

3 Things I Love About Me Today

 #1: _____

 #2: _____

 #3: _____

Daily Journal Entry:

_____

_____

_____

_____

_____

_____

_____

_____

_____

_____

_____

_____

_____

_____

_____

_____

AM Log

Date: Day: Hours of Sleep:

Morning Weight: Start Weight: Weight Lost

H2O CHECK-OFF

| 20 Ounces | 20 Ounces | 20 Ounces |
| 20 Ounces | 20 Ounces | 20 Ounces |

FOOD

LOG

Breakfast	Snack	Lunch	Snack	Dinner

PM Log

3 Things I Love About Me Today

 #1: _____

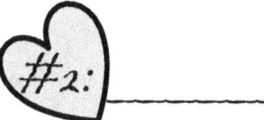 #2: _____

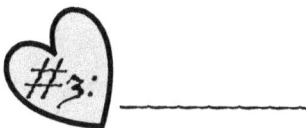 #3: _____

Daily Journal Entry:

_____

_____

_____

_____

_____

_____

_____

_____

_____

_____

_____

_____

_____

_____

_____

_____